HUMOR
AFTER THE
TUMOR

To Sara—
Wishing you
health & humor!
Love,
Patty
:)

"...Patty Gelman, invites you to join her in her year long journey through "Cancer World..."

"Roswell Park patient and breast cancer survivor, Patty Gelman, invites you to join her in her year-long journey through "Cancer World" – a journey that NO ONE wants to take! From knowing that she was from a family at very high risk for breast cancer to her diagnosis, to treatment, and finally to recovery, Patty shares her innermost fears, frustration, and joys through her e-mails to friends and family. Candidly and often with great humor, Patty recounts the enormous range of emotions that each of us has felt experiencing cancer ourselves or in a beloved family member. This book will help newly diagnosed women as well as spouses, children, and friends of patients."

Anne Gioia
Co-Founder and Chair,
Roswell Park Alliance

"This book is a very personal diary of one woman's daily physical and psychological battle against breast cancer. Patty Gelman's perspective is fresh, humorous, and self-deprecating. Her style is tremendously engaging and highly entertaining. As we travel with her along her unwanted journey of diagnosis and treatments, we gain priceless insight into the process, the toll it takes, and the successful result.

"If conquering breast cancer is at least fifty percent positive attitude, this inspirational work by a beautiful mind is a must-read for anyone facing the disease."

Clay Hamlin, Trustee
National Prostate Cancer Coalition
Philadelphia, Pa.

"A positive mind, a plan, and friends are crucial in winning the battle with cancer. Patty Gelman, while meeting the challenges of this disease, discovered a modern day strategy that replaces fear and despair with courage and optimism. Her book is pure inspiration for women coping with breast cancer."

Kenneth N. Condrell, Ph.D.
Assistant Clinical Professor
Department of Psychiatry, State University
of New York at Buffalo

"Rarely does a book come along that you wish would never end. Patty Gelman has created such a treasure. She is a fresh new voice inviting us along on her journey of overcoming breast cancer with humor, courage, and a determination that is awesome. To say this memoir is an inspiration is an understatement: anyone who has faced his or her own personal abyss of tragedy, and felt overwhelmed, must read this book; readers will be empowered by the strength of the human spirit when it says 'I can.'"

Laura Ureta Grand, M.D.
Buffalo Medical Group

"I thank Patty Gelman for allowing me to read her memoir. It is full of good humor, good sense, and good affection. I read it all within the day she gave it to me and since I know the good outcome, I am twice over pleased."

Thomas P. O'Connor, M.D., P.C.
Radiation Oncology
Western New York Medical Park

"This is a delightful chronicle of the author's journey through the morass of detection and treatment of breast cancer. It is liberally interspersed with humor; medical facts; and the important role that family, friends, and advocates played in Patty Gelman's perplexing journey. Throughout this book, the author's ability to be an active participant, along with her physicians, in making the treatment decisions, played a key role in the successful conclusion to this journey."

Robert J. Patterson, M.D.
Clinical Professor Emeritus in the
Department of Obstetrics and Gynecology
of the State University of New York at
Buffalo School of Medicine and Biomedical
Sciences. Retired Obstetrician and
Gynecologist, Retired Hospice Physician

"A husband, three children, a dog, a faulty water heater, a mother who is ill, and a diagnosis of breast cancer. That's life. Addressing it with humor, honesty, and a warm heart...that's living.

"Patty Gelman's story of her own diagnosis and treatment approaches the serious business of cancer with a hopeful and light heart. Her story is a trail guide for surviving cancer and thriving, using the resources available to each of us – love, faith, family, and friends."

Judith Brown Bryan, M.Div., C.S.W.
Spiritual Director, Candidate for Ministry,
Presbyterian Church (U.S.A)

HUMOR
AFTER THE
TUMOR

One Woman's Look at Her
Year with Breast Cancer

PATTY GELMAN

Afterword by Dr. Stephen Edge

Chair, Department of Breast and Soft Tissue Surgery, Roswell Park Cancer Institute
Professor of Surgery, State University of New York at Buffalo

Illustrations by Leslie Zemsky

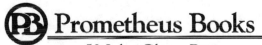

Prometheus Books

59 John Glenn Drive
Amherst, New York 14228-2119

Published 2004 by Prometheus Books

Cover photos courtesy of Mark Dellas

Inquiries should be addressed to
Prometheus Books
59 John Glenn Drive
Amherst, New York 14228–2119
VOICE: 716–691–0133, ext. 210
FAX: 716–691–0137
WWW.PROMETHEUSBOOKS.COM

11 10 09 08   7 6 5

Library of Congress Cataloging-in-Publication Data

Gelman, Patty.
    Humor after the tumor : one woman's look at her year with breast cancer / by Patty Gelman ; afterword by Stephen Edge ; illustrations by Leslie Zemsky.
        p. cm.
    ISBN 978–1–59102–218–3
    1. Gelman, Patty—Health. 2. Breast—Cancer—Patients—Biography.
I. Title.

RC280.B8G445 2003
362.196'99449'0092—dc22
[B]   2003022538

Printed in the United States on acid-free paper

Why This Book?

This book started as a series of emails, updating friends and family about the stages of my journey as I traveled through Cancer World.

After my diagnosis, messages from friends and family accumulated rapidly on my answering machine and in my computer, and emailing seemed to me the easiest way to respond. I didn't want to see people much of the time that year, nor did I want to feel like a broken record on the phone. But I knew they cared and I appreciated hearing from them. I also discovered how important writing emails became to **me**. I enjoyed recording my experiences and venting my emotions that way. Friends who had been through this before told me to keep a journal. I wrote about everything in these emails instead.

Gradually I realized that my emails were doing more than communicating with friends and family, and sustaining and entertaining me. While I was providing way too much information for some people -- my husband Warren complained about this the most -- others told me that they not only looked forward to receiving my emails, but also forwarded them to relatives, to friends, and to friends of friends. I was creating a support group. It occurred to me that others outside my personal network might benefit from reading my story.

Throughout my life, I've been lucky to have been inspired by friends and members of my family who have handled breast cancer and other major challenges in their lives with strength and humor. I saw an opportunity to pass that approach on to others. I saw an opportunity to help people whose fear of the unknown could be managed by learning from my experiences.

And so the project has grown.

Some day, with more research, we will improve our detection and even prevention of breast cancer. By offering all the royalties from this book to Roswell Park Cancer Institute in Buffalo, New York, the medical center where I received my care, I can contribute resources needed to achieve this goal. I hope to offer to all readers a story that will entertain and enlighten them. And for those readers who cope with the challenges of the disease, I hope to encourage them and to raise their spirits.

Introduction

If you want to make God laugh, make a plan.

I had a plan for my breast cancer, and it was simple. I was going to get the disease. I was going to handle it expeditiously. I was going to move on with my life.

Yes, I was going to get the disease. I had expected to do so since my mother had her first mastectomy twenty-nine years ago. My grandmother had had breast cancer before my mother, as had each of my maternal aunts as well, so it just seemed to be a matter of "when" for me instead of "if." Even after the onset of menopause moved me from being a "high risk" candidate to a more comfortable spot in the fifty percent risk group, I still figured I would get breast cancer eventually, and thus my grand plan stayed firmly in place. The specifics of the plan? An annual routine mammogram would reveal a lump the size of a pin. Early detection would indicate a double mastectomy and reconstructive surgery at the same time, and before I knew it, I'd come out with my life saved and two perky new breasts!

Fate had a different plan for me.

My routine mammogram on September 10, 2001, showed nothing, but a sonogram on the same day revealed a mass from which the doctor could not extract clear fluid. This was a cause of some concern for me, especially since I would have to wait a week for the pathology report. I didn't sleep well the night of the 10th, thinking about that eternally long week ahead of me, but on the morning of September 11th, our world changed forever and my problem became very small. Like everyone else, I spent the week riveted to the TV. Somewhere along the way, I did tell my husband, Warren, though not the rest of my family, about my situation. I told him that I would want him to share news like this with me.

We were both relieved when the pathology report came back negative. I did have to ask the woman on the phone if being negative was a positive thing. She sort of laughed. "Yes," she said, "you have no cancer." She also told me that the doctor wanted to see me in January.

On December 25, a few months later, I felt a lump. My oldest daughter, Sarah, telephoned and woke me up in bed that morning, and as I propped myself up on my elbows to talk to her, the fingers of one hand felt a lump in my armpit the size of a large grape. Quickly, I felt the other armpit for an identical lump. Finding nothing there, I made myself assume that what I'd discovered was a cyst, and first thing the next morning I called the breast clinic. Come right in, I was told, but how to do this was the question. We were in the midst of what was being called the "Snowstorm of the Century," offices were closing, and a driving ban in Buffalo had gone into effect. When I talked to my gynecologist to get her advice about what to do, she assured me that waiting until after New Year's Day was not a problem. Even if it were cancer, one week would not make a difference in any outcome.

She examined me on January 2nd. She couldn't feel the lump in my armpit until I sat up, but when she did, she recommended that I be seen by a breast surgeon and gave me the names of two of them. The first doctor could not see me for two weeks — and here I arrive at another important part of my story. My mother in Naples, Florida, had just been diagnosed with lung cancer, and I was anxious to join my sister, Cathy, from Manhattan and my brother, Harry, from Ann Arbor, who were already there with her. Waiting two weeks for an appointment with breast surgeon #1 simply wasn't going to work, and thus I was relieved when breast surgeon #2 could see me on the 8th. I'd leave for Florida the day after that, still confident that my lump was a cyst.

My middle daughter, Lisa, was a medical student at the University of Buffalo and helped us navigate all the information that was to come. She went with me to my appointment on January 8th. The surgeon couldn't feel the lump either, until again I sat up. Then, not only did he feel the lump in my armpit, but he also felt a smaller one, about the size of a pea, in my breast.

I have been grateful not only for his finding what turned out to be the primary source, but also for his request that both Lisa and I feel it as well. Doing so gave Lisa practical experience and it gave me the conviction that I would *not* have found it myself! Self-exams were never my forte, so I am sure pangs of guilt would have been overwhelming if he had pointed out something obvious. I would have been asking myself, *How could I have missed that?*

Knowing how eager I was to fly to Florida to be with my mother, he was able to schedule a surgical biopsy to remove both lumps the very next morning.

There was a downside to the arrangement. The only place available on such short notice for my little operation was an ambulatory surgery center which did not have its own pathology lab. My tissues would have to be sent to a hospital lab, and the pathology report would be delayed. The doctor would have to call Warren with the results, instead of me, since the day after the procedure, I'd be off to Florida. That was still fine with me, distracted as I was with my need to be with my mother. We had been telling her that I couldn't leave Buffalo earlier because I had a "very important meeting." Luckily she hadn't asked what sort of meeting that could possibly be, distracted as *she* was with *her* situation.

On January 9th my surgery was quick and easy. And then, on January 10th, when my bag was packed and I was ready to go (do you hear echoes of Peter, Paul and Mary?), my sister and brother called from Florida. They had decided to fly my mother to Buffalo. Good decision for everyone involved!

On January 11th I tried not to think about my pathology report while I readied the house for my mother's arrival.

Warren called. "Hi," he said. "What are you doing?"

"Just waiting here to find out if I have cancer!" I said.

His response: **"Well, you do."** A boot went into my stomach as he continued. "The doctor is glad you're still in town and wants to meet with us in his office in one hour to discuss this. He said your cancer didn't show up on the mammogram or sonogram, *which concerns him*. I'm on my way home to pick you up."

I hung up and burst into tears. That line about something concerning the doctor scared me. All I could think of was the lump in Debra Winger's armpit in *Terms of Endearment*. The phone rang again. I composed myself.

"Are you all right?" Warren asked.

"No," I said, "but you're on your way home,

right? So come home."

I hung up fast and burst into tears again.

As I've played that scene over and over in my mind, I am convinced that there is no good way to deliver bad news. You may as well just get it out and deal with it! As we drove to the doctor's office, I was already rationalizing. I had had a good life, I said to Warren, and many people had problems bigger than mine. This was a conversation he and I had had before, and I convinced both of us that I was prepared for what lay ahead.

The doctor's opinion, based on my age, family history, and attitude, was to do a bilateral mastectomy with reconstruction at the same time. We were all for it. This was, after all, my grand plan! He set up scans and tests, and also appointments for the coming week with the plastic surgeon and the oncologist who would be working with him. He also told me during my visit that ten percent of all breast cancers do not show up on mammograms. Here was information I had not known in devising that grand plan.

I was composed and tried to sound upbeat as

I called each of my daughters — Sarah, 27; Lisa, 26; and Susan, 21. It was not until I said, "I've had a good life," that the tears began to flow. Both Sarah and Susan were angry, each with the same reaction: I was the healthiest person they knew, had the healthiest lifestyle, did everything I was supposed to, so what was the point and what good did it do me? I knew immediately just what to say in response: *none of this was my fault.* With the panoply of emotions whirling around me, I could at least find some relief and comfort in this conviction.

I called my brother, Harry, with my news as he was en route with my mother to Buffalo (my sister, Cathy, had left them to return to New York), and we strategized about how to tell her about me. I suggested that he bring up the subject of her mastectomies, getting her to talk about the positive attitude she'd had at the time of each and reminiscing about how neither meant a death sentence. Harry did just this, so by the time she arrived and we told her my news, all I had to say was, "Well, it's my turn now!"

The next week was spent getting scans, x-rays, and tests and meeting with doctors. The oncologist was to be my mother's doctor as well as mine, and after he finished her examination, he talked to us about my case. Here suddenly was another curve ball thrown at my plan. Because the cancer had spread to at least one lymph node, he recommended radiation after chemotherapy, and this would preclude reconstruction at the same time as the bilateral mastectomy. Later that day we met the plastic surgeon, and she concurred with what the oncologist had told us. I would have to wait until after the radiation was finished to go back into surgery for those two perky new breasts. She did assure me, however, that eventually I'd never have to wear a bra again. I told her that that had been my plan — the plan, I added, that seemed now to be unraveling, at least in regard to the timeline I had concocted for its various parts.

On January 17th we sought a second opinion from Dr. Stephen Edge at Roswell Park Cancer Institute in Buffalo. He, too, agreed that reconstruction would have to wait. However, he disagreed about the need for a bilateral mastectomy. In his opinion, twenty years of data no longer supported a case for that course of treatment. He explained that the cancer already in my body posed a greater risk for recurrence than would any new cancer in the future; therefore he would choose to perform a lumpectomy. After that, Dr. Ellis Levine, the oncologist on his team, would attack with aggressive chemo, followed by radiation, and then either Tamoxifen or Arimidex for five years.

One factor that helped me make my decision not to have a bilateral mastectomy was this: I had always thought that without breasts, one could *not* develop breast cancer. Now I had learned that such is not necessarily the case since breast tissue can remain behind the chest wall. After days of deliberation with family and friends about this and all the other information we had gathered, we decided together that I'd go with Dr. Edge and his team at Roswell Park.

From this point on, my emails tell my story.

Sunday, January 20
7:44 A.M.

After listening to all
the options and opinions and
variables, I've decided to have a
lumpectomy with further lymph node
excision at Roswell Park, with Dr. Edge, on
February 1. After a few weeks, his team will start
me on chemotherapy for eight sessions followed
by radiation. The prediction is that I will feel
wiped out for a part of each month and my hair
will fall out. In September, or October, I'll be all
finished! I'll be doing physical therapy shortly
after my surgery to regain full range of motion
with my left arm. Dr. Edge made a very
convincing case for this approach, saying that
the latest scientific and medical data does not
support a more radical, aggressive approach
(i.e., bilateral mastectomy). I face a greater risk
from the cancer that is in my body right now
than from any that could develop in the future,
and that is what they will attack with the
treatments.

The one factor that may change our minds is

my genetic make-up. Therefore, I'm having my blood drawn on Wednesday, at Roswell, and sent to a genetic laboratory for "DNA sequencing" to determine if I have a mutation in one of the identified "breast cancer genes." We will hear the results of the tests in a week, which will help us decide which surgery to choose: lumpectomy or bilateral mastectomy. If I do have that mutation, it puts me in a ninety percent risk category for recurrence, in which case Dr. Edge would be more inclined to suggest a bilateral mastectomy. Having said that, he insists that the final decision will rest squarely on our shoulders. So a little more waiting for that decision, but *much* more understanding! I think my explanation is accurate; I'll run it by Dr. Lisa to make sure.

As for my mother, she is happy as a clam. She's still in the hospital being tested inside and out, up and down, and feels comfortable now that she's on oxygen and steroids. The goal is to keep her comfortable; therefore she'll be going through radiation and chemo too! She will probably come home Tuesday and start her treatments once a day, everyday. She'll be tired and lose her hair. She says she wants a blonde wig!

Maybe whatever cancer she has can be treated, but we are assuming it cannot and, as she keeps saying, we are making the best of what time she has left. She has not lost her micro-management skills or her sense of humor!

Love, Patty

Tuesday, January 22
9:58 A.M.

I feel good. Thanks. I even slept well over the weekend! Last night was back to the 3:00 A.M. wake-up. So I went upstairs and changed all the linens from the weekend's visitors: Cathy, Charley, my ten-year-old nephew, and Susan, who came home from the University of Vermont, where she's a junior. I made up the beds for my brother, Harry, and whoever else lands here this weekend!

I had been worried that Susan would use my mother's condition and mine as an excuse to become distracted from her schoolwork. It was wonderful to see her and be convinced that she's got her act together and she's "not going to blow it now" (her words). She also loves working part-time at a day care center and just emailed me the following note: *"I thought it was important to inform my professors about what's up in my life. In the case of a funeral, I can make a quick phone call and there will be no surprises or huge problem finding a sub for me. Also, it makes life a little easier knowing that they know.*

Gotta go to class now. See, I'm focused."

My mother "Mia" has set a tone that has made it easier for all the grandchildren to deal with the situation. Yesterday, my brother's wife, Jan, sent an email to everyone. She said that when Harry returned from Buffalo, he was sitting at the table eating blueberries with his ten-year-old twins, Ethan and Jeremy. He told them that Mia has cancer, she's quite ill, and at some point she may die. They both listened and nodded. Then Jeremy asked, "Dad, are there any more blueberries?" My mother loved that!

Warren came up with a spontaneous plan to go to Toronto Saturday to see *Mamma Mia* and I'm looking forward to that. My brother will come from Ann Arbor to be with my mother while we're gone. Spontaneity will have to be the operative word for a while. No long-term planning until my mother meets her fate. No tears here, please; she is instructing everyone to be cheerful and realistic and focus on the great life she has had.

She has been providing us with precise directions for her cremation and wants the memorial service to be for both her and my father, since we never had one up here when he died in Naples six years ago.   Sarah was unpacking for her, as my mother sat in her chair issuing directives, when Sarah picked up a very heavy case and said, "Mia, it feels like there's a brick in here!"   My mother said, "Oh, that's Grandpa. Put him in the closet until it's time for us to be buried together! *Don't forget him!*" She even dictated what she wants us to say at her memorial service.

She just called to say that the doctor said she could go home today, so I'll be picking her up after my meeting at Roswell this morning. They'll send oxygen and a wheelchair to our house and she'll start her radiation tomorrow at the Essjay Road office: once a day, every day. She says she feels okay as she waits for the other shoe to drop. No one predicts when that will be.

Love, Patty

Thursday, January 31
6:21 P.M.

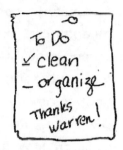

To Do
✓ clean
— organize
Thanks
warren!

The results of the genetic analysis came back today. Sarah, Lisa, Warren, and I planned to be gathered at home at 5:00 P.M. when Dr. Edge and the genetic counselor from Roswell were scheduled to call us. When the call came in, each one of us was on a phone so we could hear the report. I'd say it was a collective holding of our breath as we heard, "The official interpretation of this result is that this is a genetic variant of *uncertain significance*." I was expecting something more like, "You've got the mutation!" or "You don't!"

We all asked for an explanation. The counselor went on to read that "it is *suspected*, but *not yet proven*, that this variant is more likely to be a variation of limited clinical significance rather than associated with cancer susceptibility," based on data collected so far. There are future studies being planned and if the "contribution of this variant to the relative risk of breast or ovarian cancer can be established, then a revised report will be issued." In the meantime, with the information at hand, we all agreed that I did not appear to be in a greater risk category; therefore we opted for a lumpectomy instead of a bilateral mastectomy. Dr. Edge will be doing further lymph node excision as well.

I have to be at Roswell tomorrow morning at 7:30 and surgery will be around 9:00 A.M. Dr. Edge expects that I'll be in the hospital for two or three days and Warren is taking my crash course: *"HOW TO PLEASE PATTY BY PUTTING THINGS IN THEIR PLACES!"*

I appreciate all the helpful advice from those of you who've been through this, especially from my college friend who not only had a bilateral mastectomy and reconstruction four years ago, but also works for an information management company in the Health Division. She's the project director of several health information contracts. Her two primary contracts are with the National Cancer Institute and the National Center for Complementary and Alternative Medicine. She has been and will continue to be a wonderful resource and an inspiration for me!

Thank you all for your good wishes!

Love, Patty

Thursday, February 7
7:52 P.M.

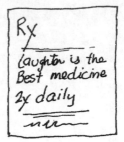

Rx
laughter is the
Best medicine
2x daily
nu

I felt fine after the surgery and devoured the meal that arrived the first evening. Sarah told me I looked as if I'd been hit by a truck, and I did throw up the meal as soon as everyone left. But I felt great by the next day and went home.

At our appointment with Dr. Edge today, he was happy to tell us that the pathology report indicated all of the twelve lymph nodes he removed were clear and I had clean margins in the breast. So our next stop is to the oncologist, Dr. Levine, on Monday. He will tell us when he will start the chemotherapy. I'll give a detailed report to you all after that meeting.

Meanwhile, I have a draining tube connected to a grenade-shaped plastic reservoir. The tube drains from under my left armpit, where the nodes were removed, and each day I measure and empty the fluid that collects in it. Dr. Edge didn't want to remove the tube until I have less fluid draining, which he predicts will be when I'm back to Roswell on Monday for the Dr. Levine visit. That means a few more uncomfortable nights with the help of the pain pills to help me fall back to sleep after each time I roll over; but it only hurts at level three or four out of ten. As I've mentioned to some of you already, we know there's a problem in this house when *Warren* is the best sleeper.

At least my days are easy and I am continuously grateful that the lumps weren't on my right side, because I'm right-handed! As Warren arrived this afternoon to take me to Roswell, I had no problem, before we left, following behind his trail of food and mud and cleaning it all up with the pain-free arm. I'm in heaven: you all cook for us and I get to clean up and remain in some sort of control!

There's no point in predicting when I'll be starting chemo; we'll know that on Monday. My mother is feeling and looking so good that her doctor wants to start her on some mild chemo right now, while she's having the radiation. He was visibly surprised that she looked so strong. She says that she's sure he's just trying to make her look *worse*! Dr. Lisa is now working on convincing her that the side effects will be mild if there are any at all. We all agree that we're having too much fun here to have him mess things up with nausea or hot flashes! We'll keep you posted.

My sister, Cathy, and her son, Charley, are coming to Buffalo again this weekend from New York, and Susan is coming from Burlington. Susan feels out of the loop being away at college. Sarah and Lisa are able to see us every day, which is especially great for my mother and why it was such a good decision to bring her up here from Naples.

And, while she is looking forward to this weekend, she insists that nobody should disrupt one's life because of her situation. My brother-in-law Jayson made her feel comfortable with the plan when he told her he would be out of town anyway, so it was a perfect time for Cathy's visit to Buffalo. Since we know we'll be laughing most of the time, it will be a perfect chance to try out these new little pills and watch for negative results in the midst of all the positive distractions.

More later. All the best.

Love, Patty

Wednesday, February 11
10:18 P.M.

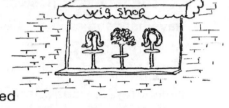

As Dr. Ellis Levine introduced himself, he apologized for what he called the *barbaric* way he was obliged to treat me and regretted what my body was going to have to go through. He said he hoped that some day the drugs he uses now could be replaced by better strategies! Then he explained everything to Warren and to me very clearly, with the aid of a writing board on the wall and all kinds of time for answers to our questions.

Warren was more interested in the statistics and I was more interested in the logistics. As soon as I am healed completely from my surgery, Dr. Edge will give Dr. Levine clearance to start the chemotherapy. I have an appointment with them both on February 21. Assuming that I'm cleared for take-off, Dr. Levine will book my first treatment. It would probably be within those following two weeks; but he and Dr. Edge emphasize that there is *no rush!* Once I start, I would go for eight sessions of intravenous chemo at Roswell. There will be twenty days between each session, so it will take a total of six months.

During the first four sessions, I will be receiving a combination of Cytoxin and Adriamycin, taking approximately an hour for each session. During the last four sessions, I'll be on Taxol, which will take a total of four hours each session. After the six months of chemo, I'll have radiation for six or eight weeks, then go on hormonal therapy (probably Tamoxifen or, I hope, some alternative with fewer negative side effects!). Hormonal Therapy is used to keep cancer cells from receiving the hormones they need to grow. **It is not the same as Hormone Replacement Therapy!**

So you can see that while Warren was more interested in survival-rate statistics, I was more into *Where do I go and what will you do to me?* I will lose my hair for sure, he said, and I might be nauseous, might be wiped-out for part of each 20-day cycle, and might have mouth sores. So all of you people who have been determined to fatten me up must now put on the brakes!

Warren, who has never noticed my changing hairstyles in 30 years, is passing on to me all kinds of wig information he's receiving from friends and clients. I thought it was particularly noteworthy that he wanted to know what I thought of the idea of shaving my head at the first sign of hair loss. A friend of his suggested I do that since it worked out so well for his wife when she did it. It happens that I did shave the head of a friend of mine when her hair started to fall out in annoying clumps; I had convinced her at the time that it would be much more comfortable, which it was! But aren't we all thinking the same thing here: doesn't he just want another bald head to match his?

He's thrilled about the recommendation that I avoid large groups of people in confined spaces when my blood count is low and my immune system is compromised, to avoid infection. In summary, I'll be tired, bald, and anti-social occasionally, for the next eight months. That's not really much of a problem at all, except for the unknown condition of my mother.

My friend Michele May, who is very close to my mother, came over to give my mother a haircut the other night. My mother was ecstatic and insists that it's *the best haircut she's ever had in her whole life!*

To be perfectly honest, we feel very lucky that you all make this so easy and fun! We do not feel that we are in this alone. So we'll take one day at a time and continue to *make the best of it!*

Love, Patty

Thursday, February 28
4:42 P.M.

Millicent & Herman

My mother had a difficult time catching her breath in the early morning hours of Sunday, Feb. 17. She was scared, but didn't ring the little bell I'd given her until 4:00 A.M. because she didn't want to wake us up! Hospice has been on board from the time she arrived here, and we called them to find out how to give her relief. The bag of drugs they'd provided had everything we needed to help her, but it was clear to all of us that she'd taken a significant turn for the worse.

This was a woman who daily devoured the *New York Times* as enthusiastically as Warren reads our sports section! And she especially loved the *Sunday Times*! But when it arrived that Sunday morning, she looked at it and said, "Ugh, that looks like so much work! There must be something really wrong with me!" She adored Maureen Dowd's column, so I read it aloud to her while she lay back in her recliner and listened with her eyes closed.   She slept most of the day and proclaimed that she did not want to go through another night like the last one and wanted to go to the Hospice facility.

The plan was that she would be in there for what Hospice calls a *Respite Stay*, while we found a nurse who would live with us during the nights. While the nurse from Hospice explained that a *Respite Stay* can be up to five days, my mother turned to Lisa and quietly quipped, *"I have up to five days to die."*

We left her there on Sunday night, very happy, comfortable, and quiet, enjoying some chicken soup. As we were leaving, she asked me to find the figure skating on TV and we all said good night.   Unfortunately, she had another difficult night there.

When I arrived in the morning, she was either sleeping or very doped up. She did show her personality for a moment when I asked her if she wanted any of my warm vanilla soy milk, and she made a funny face and gesture like: *get that stuff away, no, no!* But other than that, she was in another world. The doctor told me that she probably wouldn't live more than another day. I called Cathy, Harry, Susan, and Marlane (the wonderful woman who had been helping us during the days), and we were all in her room when she took her last breath the following morning.

We are sad as we miss her and happy as we remember her cheerful outlook. Those of you who were able to be at her memorial service heard that she *dictated* exactly what she wanted us to say because she was afraid we wouldn't get it right! For you out-of-towners, here it is:

The best years of her life were with Herman, and their life revolved completely around their three "magnificent" children and six "equally fantastic" grandchildren. (She insisted we use those adjectives!) After Herman died, her happiest moments were in the company of her family.

She always said that when her time came, there were to be no tears or sorrow because she had a wonderful life. Fifty-one years with my father and her only regret was that she could not attend her own funeral. But she did her best to arrange everything happening here today.

Her philosophy of life was this: we only go through one time, so we'd better appreciate what we have and make the best of everything that happens to us.

Then, honoring her wishes, everyone went to The Buffalo Club to *"celebrate Herman and Millicent's life."*

I am fortified by the memory of her responding the same way every time I brought up the possibility that we might lament her passing. She said, "Don't waste your time missing me. Turn your attention to your children."

As most parents do, Warren's parents, Jack and Barbara, and mine supplied us with wisdom throughout our lives. My mother always instructed us to learn from life's lessons and move forward. During those last days, she seemed to delight in a favorite line from Shakespeare's *The Tempest*: **"What is past is prologue!"** She repeatedly chanted it, lying back in her recliner with eyes closed.

We feel lucky to have the memories and we're counting on our luck continuing!

Wishing you the same.

Love, Patty

Friday, March 1
9:00 A.M.

I start chemo on Monday, March 4. I might have nausea for the first few days and I will be "hugging the couch" for the first four days; then I'll feel fine. I'll have a higher risk of infection from day #10 to day #14, then I'll feel like Wonder Woman until day #21 when we start the whole cycle over again.

I will have to have my blood count taken every week, and if I spike a fever, I am supposed to call immediately. Dr. Levine made this point emphatically saying, "*If your temperature is 101 at 3 A.M., I want my phone ringing by 3:05 AM! Do not wait until morning, thinking that you don't want to bother me. We'll probably want to hook you up to IV antibiotics in the hospital to fight the infection.*" One has to appreciate a doctor who offers that level of comfort!

My hair will start to fall out on day #7, and I am ready with my plan to look like Katie Couric. We are going to Toronto on March 9, to have dinner with friends and see Jerry Seinfeld. I have an appointment that afternoon to cut my hair very short (or shave it all off, depending on how much has fallen out by then) and walk out of the salon with the hair I've always wanted!

I am keeping my focus on the big picture and appreciating all the concern! Sarah encouraged me to use the "chemo card" whenever I can, so I tried it out on Warren last night when I asked him *again* if we could invest in a giant hot water tank. I explained that it would allow me to take longer showers. He said no.

I'll just have to rely on him, the dogs, and these wonderful hot flashes to warm me up.

Stay warm yourselves.

Love, Patty

Monday, March 4
7:45 P.M.

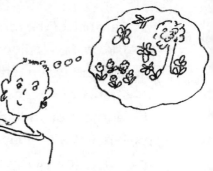

Warren took me to my first chemo session today, and everything went well. I am waiting to feel nausea, but Dr. Levine's assistant, Sharon, loaded me up with anti-nausea meds and sent me home with more to take for the next four days, so I feel fine. I was worried that maybe the chemo wasn't working because I felt so good, but Dr. Lisa was over here a minute ago and made me feel better by assuring me that I'll feel worse tomorrow. I plan to be sleepy until Thursday when the nausea period will have passed!

This morning I received a good report from the physical therapist, who said I was doing well and should have full range of motion in my arm and shoulder in a few months. I convinced him that I didn't deserve his praise for doing the simple reaching and stretching exercises he'd assigned because I'm 5' 1" and forced to reach and stretch for almost everything.

Because of the removal of lymph nodes, I am at risk of developing lymphedema, which is a permanent, irreversible swelling of the arm and chest area that sometimes develops after either the surgery or radiation. Therefore, in order to prevent it, I will always have to take extra care of my arm by avoiding cuts, blood draws, injections, blood pressure straps, and heavy lifting on that side. Most activities are good exercise and the PT said he *saw no reason why I couldn't play golf this summer!*

Let's pause here and allow a moment for a good laugh for those of you who have seen me on a golf course. The rest of you will appreciate the joke when you understand that I would love to someday rise to the level of "horrible golfer". Right now, Warren says what I do on a course cannot be called "golf."

My next move is to enroll in a "Look Good, Feel Better" class. There I will learn how to paint eyebrows and put makeup on a very pale face! A friend sent me a wonderful book, *Breast Cancer, There and Back* by Jami Bernard. It's a helpful guide and filled with humor. In it she suggests ways to redirect my focus from too much worry by *thinking about things like mapping out the perfect garden or making a mental catalog of your dog's body language!*

I am looking forward to meeting the wig lady in Toronto this weekend. She is planning to cut my hair short and fit the wig to that. We've agreed that Warren's time will be much better spent watching a couple of youth hockey games up there that day. I'm reminded of the time I came home with a full perm, and he never noticed a difference. He's not the guy you want offering opinions on wig selection. We had a Cocker Spaniel for sixteen years, and I wondered how it was that whenever Max came back from the groomer, Warren would arrive home from work and always greet him with enthusiasm and tell him how great he looked. I finally said that my feelings were a little hurt that he *never* noticed my changing hairstyles over the years, but he *always* noticed Max's. He said, "They put a bow on him."

***

About my mother, I miss her deeply, but all the cancer conversation has been a distraction from the heartache, and vice versa. So I feel less grief, and less worry for *now*. If I start throwing up, that deal's off!

Love, Patty

Sunday, March 10
10:01 A.M.

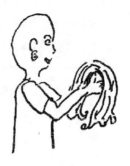

Well, it is for real now. I have cancer. Once my head was shaved, there was no denying it! That part was actually fun; there have been many times when I have been tempted to do this in fits of desperation with styling. As Sartre said, *"Life begins on the far side of despair."* Only my life has to wait six months!

I'm sorry to report that the next part was not as successful. I don't know which was more hilarious, my wig or Jerry Seinfeld! He really was funny, and distracted me from my hair for the better part of a couple of hours. However, seated in the first row, I was at times self-conscious and paranoid, convinced that everyone was staring at my wig, and even worried that at any moment he was going to make a joke about it!

I will cut it and work with it and ... never leave my house. I look terrible in hats, and I tried on scarves, but looked too much like Aunt Jemima.

So I'll see y'all in September!

Love, Patty

Wednesday, March 13
6:30 P.M.

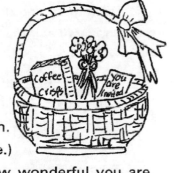

Hello,   everyone!
(Sounds like Karl Haas on
the classical music station.
Think of his soothing voice.)
You all need to know how wonderful you are.
You make it really easy to have cancer: dinners,
Coffee Crisps, errands, flowers, phone calls,
cards, spa gift certificates, more Coffee Crisps,
dog-sitting, invitations My friend Shelley is
convincingly disappointed if I don't have a long
supermarket list for her every week!

A friend of Sarah and Lisa, Jordan Griffin,
sent me a poem he wrote and gave me
permission to share it with you:

What will they say?

What will they say
When they see that I am so thin?
They will say how strong you look.

What will they say

49

When they see how pale I am?
They will say that you are fair.

What will they say
When they see I have no hair?
They will say you are exotic.

What will they say
When they see I have scars?
They will say you are a woman.

What will they say
When they see that I am afraid?
They will say that you give them hope.

Why?
Because you are beautiful.

This may be Cancer World, but it's also heaven! My Coffee Crisp inventory must be over forty and that's important for a reserve supply because one never knows when Tom Ridge will have to call a red security alert and the bridges to Canada will be really backed up. (Coffee Crisps are sold only in Canada.)   Not to make light of September 11: watching the memorials on Monday, weren't we all sad yet grateful to be alive?!

I do feel terrific. The steroids made sleeping impossible for a few nights and that bothered me, so Dr. Levine's assistant, Sharon, agreed to let me try to go it without them next time. I might miss the super strength however! I have rearranged the furniture in two rooms already, and I have my eye on a shelving unit that begs to be moved in Susan's room. I'm trying to create more of a Bed and Breakfast look in there and less of a sorority house atmosphere. With this compulsion to move furniture, I decided to reread my book on Feng Shui; it would be a shame to discover, once the steroids wear off, that I've put everything in the wrong spaces, when I'll be too weak to do anything about it! And we need all the *balance and harmony* we can achieve around here! I do feel strong now; it is all I can do to resist picking up my adorable dog Kambel, but he's a Golden Retriever and these steroids must have their limits.

Last night I noticed that a spotlight was out on the family room ceiling. No problem: I moved sections of the couch, dragged the coffee table out of the way, hauled in the ladder, and changed the bulb. Warren was on the other part of the couch and gave me the dreaded "look." That was not because he was worried I'd slip a disk or get lymphedema, but because I was bothering him while *JAG* was on TV. The honeymoon's definitely over and thank goodness he's back to his old self. For dinner he grilled steaks outside. I said mine was delicious and asked how he made it so crunchy. He looked over and said, "Oh, I dropped one in the mud and I must not have wiped it all off." Obviously he's not too worried about my low blood count and vulnerability to infection!

Many of you have been asking about my wig. It seems to be taking on a life of its own. Up until today, every time I tried it on it reminded me of "Cousin It" in *The Addams Family*: all hair and little legs coming out of the bottom. It did go out today, with a hat to keep the long hair out of my eyes, and tomorrow it's going to ride my head to the wonderful man at Capello's who will cut it and make me more comfortable. That way my wig and I will both get out more!

To those of you who say you want to talk to me or see me, remember back to how nasal my voice sounds and how long it takes me to get to a point. I remember eyes glazing over, or words like "Tick, tock", or "Is there an end to this story?" I once put my sister to sleep, and when I suggested to my mother that it was probably because I hadn't really known what I'd been talking about, my mother said, "Sometimes people fall asleep even when you **do** know what you're talking about!"

So I think these emails are great. Thank you again for showering me with attention. I love hearing from you. And believe me, you're better off thinking of Karl Haas's voice as you read these emails, and feeling soothed!

Love, Patty

Thursday, March 14
5:18 P.M.

You have been very worried about my wig, so here is a wonderful wig report. Joe Freitas, at Capello on Transit Rd., is a warm, friendly guy, in addition to being trained in the art of cutting and styling wigs. He knows what women with wigs want, and what to tell them about maintenance. He's also very sensitive to how they feel about losing hair and/or going through treatments. I asked him why he didn't market himself through Roswell and he said he simply wouldn't be able to handle the demand. He used to work at Roswell a couple of days a week many years ago, but he became too busy to fit it in.

I tell you all this because word-of-mouth is the only way people will find him. So if you ever know of someone else who needs him, you'll have helpful information. I love the cut he gave my wig. I think it still looks like a wig, but it makes me feel much more comfortable out in the world.

You keep saying you want to see me, so let me describe myself: with the wig I look the same as ever. As soon as I enter my house, however, I rip it off and have a gray brush cut, or a little green hat if it's chilly. Because it's St. Patrick's week, and I'm a theme dresser from way back, I am wearing nothing but green tops or a black watch sweater, a black watch plaid jacket, a green scarf, green socks and jade earrings. With my little head, large ears, and all this green, I'd say I look like a leprechaun!

Speaking of green, Warren has given the green light to the bigger hot water tank. Oh dear, there are only six months left for me to keep playing the "chemo card"! Not only that, he arrived home last night with dinner and *roses*! I asked, "Who are you and what have you done with Warren?" The truth is, if he keeps this up he will deprive all of us of good material to laugh at!

Hope you all have delicious corned beef and cabbage!

Love, Patty

Sunday, March 17
5:45 A.M.

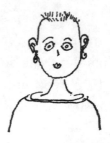

Now and then, especially during the first week of my treatment cycle, I did feel alone and afraid, especially when I found out that the effects will be cumulative, increasing with each treatment. Lisa assures me that the length of time for the ill effects stays the same, thank goodness, so it will always be just one queasy week each cycle. Most of the time I am loving the attention and allowing you all to believe I am helpless, as people offer to do everything for me. I realize this, too, shall pass and I am prepared to make the adjustment back to reality in September, when you will all be posing the appropriate and predictable, popular question, "Patty who?"

Right now, these email reports and banter are helpful for me, especially when I can't sleep; and while I am glad they are entertaining for you, I believe that turning them into a book, as many of you have suggested, is a bit of a stretch. Nevertheless, thanks for making me feel so smart and talented. I was thinking about taking my SAT's again, just one more time! I know I could bring my scores up. My IQ feels much higher than in high school. I would have to take them at 3 o'clock in the morning, however, because that's when I'm most alert! It's probably not the mind but the *miles*, as they say!

I'm so smart that I may have figured out a way to avoid buying a bigger water heater after all — I moved the energy saver dial to "hot." I would like to have a "quick recovery" option for the heater (as well as for myself, for that matter!).

Cathy and Charley are coming in this morning for a week, while my brother-in-law Jayson is away. We will have fun laughing and playing with dogs! Now my head and Charley's look exactly the same. I still have a brush cut; no hair has fallen out yet. Most people like to rub my head just as we always do to Charley's. The only person who *refuses* to feel it is Warren, who keeps saying, when approached, *"NO! NO! I do NOT want to feel it. I had hair exactly like that for twenty-six years; I know exactly what it feels like!"* The poor guy sounds nostalgic.

It seems a shame to waste the green light from Warren for the water heater. If we're not buying that, I wonder if I could get "house credit" and use it for a loveseat in the living room instead. There are not enough places for people to sit in there and Warren's response is, "Let people stand." He's the host with the most.

Speaking of hosting a party, we plan to have a big party to thank all of you for being so wonderful. As I said earlier, most of the time I feel caught up in the arms of friendship and family and will be forever grateful. I can't predict when the party will be though, because I refuse to entertain without eyebrows.

Love, Patty

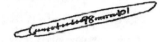

I wanted to let you know that I'm in the hospital (Roswell). On Friday morning I had a minor raw throat, so I called Nurse Sharon who put me on Cipro. By Sunday night I had a fever of 101 and my doctor wanted me in here to pump antibiotics into me through an IV. The good news is that I had time to finish a delicious dinner of corned beef and cabbage, cooked and brought over by my Uncle Sammy and Aunt Rose. I'd been taking my temp all day, watching it climb, and wondering why the Cipro wasn't working. So the truth is that I felt safer at that point being in here.

During the first night I did have a slight scare. My head started to feel like it was on fire and the nurse said my face and body were bright red. Even after she gave me some Benadryl, which gave me immediate relief, one aide said that I was still glowing in the dark! It turns out that I had what is known as "Red Man's Syndrome," a reaction to one of the antibiotics, Vancomycin. After the nurse told me that, I spent the better part of the night nervously measuring each breath, hoping with each one that there would be another breath to follow, and grateful that it wasn't called "*Dead* Man's Syndrome".

My neutrifils count is at zero and I can't go home until it's back up to 500. (Neutrifils fight bacterial infection.) Dr. Levine predicts that will be Friday or later, and we're all hoping I can stay on schedule for my next treatment on Monday. Lisa's laptop will keep me busy, as I write to and answer all of you, and I have a good book.

I feel fine.

Love, Patty

Thursday, March 21
4:41 AM

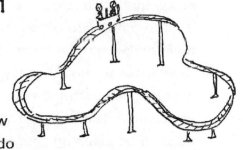

Hi, honey, I'm home! I just wanted to let you know I'm home and I do feel fine. My count is up and my temp is normal and I am on schedule for round #2 on Monday. My friend Ellen will be in town and she will take me. I was given a solution to swish around my mouth for sore gums, which were also swollen for a while. I had read that my gums might become swollen and my *teeth might feel loose.*

One night in the hospital, I was awakened by the sore gums and I started to wonder if I'd lose my teeth instead of my hair, since that seemed to remain intact! I wondered if my hair wasn't going to fall out after all and I had a brush cut for nothing! So — drum roll here — I pulled it and a little clump of little stubs appeared in my fingertips! I was so excited and gratified that no one had made an unfortunate miscalculation. I entertained myself for a while pulling my hair out, then swished some solution in my mouth and went back to sleep.

The plan for the next round of chemo is to give me Neupogen, a shot I will give myself for seven days starting Tuesday, which will boost the white blood cells and help me avoid infection in the future. The side effect: sore bones. But I hope to be sleeping through week #1, as I was last time, and not feeling a thing!

I do not miss my mother right now at all. She would have been so worried about me if she had seen all these side effects. Believe me, they're not as bad as they look, but no one would be able to convince a mother of that. I do believe there is some grand plan, or she really did control her fate, because I don't know if I would have been able to maintain my sense of humor through this if I had to watch her suffering a slow, painful death at the same time. We all felt that she checked out when she did to make it easier on all of us. Now, my biggest worry is *who's wiping the dogs' muddy feet*? Actually, I arrived home last night to a clean and tidy house, thanks to Susan (and a little to Cathy) who was well aware of how great that would make me feel, and it did!

On we go with our journey through Cancer World. What a ride! I don't think I'll ever need to go on another roller coaster again! I think one reason for my passion for roller coasters was the otherwise calm and controlled life I led. I was one of the many people who were heartbroken when the Comet left Crystal Beach Amusement Park, on the Canadian lakeshore near Buffalo. Susan and I found it in Glens Falls on our way to Vermont a few years ago, and we rode it four times in a row. It wasn't the same without Lake Erie below us, but it was fun, and I'm glad I finally rode the giant one at Darien Lake. That one had the highest drop I've ever experienced! I rode it twice in a row but don't have a full memory of the second time because I passed out briefly in the middle of the ride.

I read that an old person should not ride roller coasters because the spongy part around an older person's brain becomes hard and not able to cushion the impact as the brain bangs around on the fast descents! I probably read that in an AARP magazine.

Please appreciate the all-purpose friendship here; not only do I offer information about

Cancer World, but I also offer glimpses into the world of the aging! Believe me, the old brain, coupled with all that excitement during that one suspense-filled night in the hospital when I was wondering if I was going to be able to continue to *breathe*, makes it easy to retire from roller coasters!

This is all the excitement I can handle! The week when I was supposed to feel like Wonder Woman turned into "I wonder what else will happen?" As long as the doctors and Lisa aren't worried, neither am I.

Love, Patty

Wednesday, March 27
4:07 P.M.

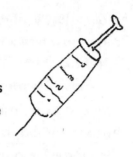

This is a test to see if this letter goes through. We're now hooked up to Adelphia cable instead of AOL.

Yesterday was round #2 and all went well. My friend Ellen kept me company and Warren stopped in to tell me that I was probably scaring all the people in the waiting room with my bald head. I had thought it was sort of like a nudist colony, where everyone was there for the same purpose and no one noticed exposed places anymore! I guess I'd better look for a lightweight spring cap! I do now have two good wigs. Cathy brought a great one for me from New York, but they are not as comfortable as a bald head.

The doctors have prescribed Neupogen, which I will inject myself starting tomorrow for a week. I have chosen to inject it into my thigh because it's a *large* target. The Neupogen is for the purpose of boosting my white blood cells. If I do land in the hospital next week, I will now know to remind them to drip the Vancomycin more slowly and give me the Benadryl before the drip starts, in order to avoid "Red Man's Syndrome"!

I love hearing from you, especially on the other side of midnight, when I'll probably be awake. Although this time we opted to eliminate the steroids, so maybe I'll sleep better and leave the furniture alone.

Love, Patty

(The following email was written with no memory of the previous one. This is a clear illustration of the mind-numbing power of those anti-nausea drugs.)

Thursday, March 28
3:25 P.M.

The second round of chemo went according to plan, even with a three-hour delay, one we've come to expect. Ellen went with me and we filled the time with books, food, articles, and a visit from Warren, who told me that I should wear a hat in the waiting room because I might be scaring the other patients.

I had always thought of Roswell along the same lines as a nudist colony, everyone there for the same purpose! I'll start looking for spring caps to satisfy Warren. He should be used to it from home where he and I look like twins now! I do have *two* good wigs; Cathy brought me one from New York and I have the first one from Toronto, so when I have to be covered, I'm all set.

I have been sleeping most of the time this week. These anti-nausea drugs do the trick. Once a day, I give myself a shot of Neupogen to boost the white blood count. I aim for my thigh, a nice *big* target.

I love hearing from you, especially on the other side of midnight, although this time we opted to eliminate the steroids. So maybe I'll sleep better and leave the furniture alone!

Have a Happy Easter and Happy Passover.

Love, Patty

Sunday, March 31
10:32 A.M.

It's Easter Sunday and I need a bonnet! Ellen says I remind her of *My Favorite Martian*. Images also come to mind of *Star Trek* or *Casper the Friendly Ghost*. Warren, taking his characteristic position of always looking out for the other guy, insists that I will make other people uncomfortable if I leave the house like this without a hat or wig. So this week I'll be on a mission to find a spring hat! The wigs are okay, but I think a hat will feel better.

It was a good decision to omit the steroids this round because I have been sleeping through every night like a log! Even though Passover began on Wednesday, Cousin Carol postponed our Seder to Friday when I was drug-free and not nauseated. She presented a wonderful meal and I especially appreciated the matzoh ball soup, a swell stomach soother! I am queasy now and then but satisfied that I don't have to rely on any drugs. If everything goes according to the last pattern, I'll be feeling great in a day or two. I have been giving myself a shot each day of

Neupogen to keep my count up, so this time I should sail from day #10 through #14 without incident.

Sorry about the email that repeated the same stuff as the one on the previous day. I had no memory of doing that. Now you see why I want to remain drug-free. Happy Passover and Happy Easter! I just thought of another seasonal image for my head: an *egg*!

Love, Patty

Wednesday, April 3
4:41 P.M.

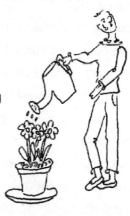

We had an interesting episode last night. I was awakened by excruciating pain that was throbbing in my lower back. I assumed I'd been sleeping in an awkward position and spent almost twenty minutes changing positions and trying to stretch it out. On the floor with legs tucked up, legs tucked under, sitting up — nothing worked. I found the only position in which I could feel any relief was *standing up!* Unfortunately it was 2:00 A.M. I didn't dare take anything for it without calling the on-call doctor first. She was puzzled until I mentioned that during the afternoon, I had just given myself my last shot of Neupogen. She gave an enlightened sigh and said it was probably a side effect from that. I was to take three Motrin and wait for up to an hour for some relief.

I had been worried all week that I might not have been giving myself the shots correctly, especially since I had experienced no bone pains all week. Therefore I was glad the Neupogen was working and I busied myself with activities around the house that I could do standing up!

I did laundry, plant watering, and standing at my desk, reading and writing back to your emails! Aren't I lucky I'm short? Thank you, thank you to the people who wrote to me in the evening since it really made the time go fast! From now on, I'm not going to check my emails after dinner in order to have something to do if I'm looking for activity in the middle of the night!

Lisa's dog, Timber, was sleeping at our house, as he often does. By the time I felt better, Warren and the two dogs were sound asleep again, with Timber, a ninety-pound Labrador Retriever, sprawled with his head on my pillow. I wedged myself in and spent the next two hours between Timber and the edge of the bed, with his head and mine sharing the pillow. I thought of that scene in *The Godfather (Part 1)* with the horse's head! At least there was no blood, and Timber was definitely breathing; he even sneezed once right in my face!

They were all so deep into their sleep that I

didn't want to cause a commotion by trying to move Timber. He and Warren were even snoring in harmony for a while. Now that I've experienced so many sleepless nights, I'm able to witness that Warren *does* sleep. My guess is that for all these years, he's been using that line about "a sleeping problem" in order to avoid or escape from parties early!

Sharon, Dr. Levine's assistant, called today to explain that indeed I had experienced the predicted bone pain about which she had warned me. The good news is that the Neupogen is doing its job, expanding the bone marrow as it stimulates the white blood cells. As the bone marrow expands, it causes pain. The even better news is that the first cycle is usually the worst and it will be less uncomfortable from now on. And the *great* news is: because the Neupogen is working, she is sure my white count will stay up; I will avoid infection and stay out of the hospital!

It might be gloomy outside, but this is a good day! So how was **your** day, dear?

Love, Patty

Tuesday, April 9
5:11 P.M.

Aren't we all glad the weather is warming up? The Neupogen worked; my count is staying up and my bone marrow is expanded and staying that way, so I am hopeful that I won't be feeling any more back pain during future cycles!

While my bone marrow is expanded, my brain will be "contracted"! I just read that Ativan, one of the drugs I take to suppress nausea during week #1, induces temporary memory loss! My book calls it "Milk of *Amnesia*"! Luckily it is temporary, lasting only the first week of each cycle, so next week I'll be smart and avoid scheduling any computer lessons or writing any updates.

Last time, I tried listening to my computer tutor and taking pages of notes, only to feel nauseated towards the end of the lesson. I forgot everything he was trying to teach me. My notes meant nothing to me later. The only thing I was successful in *downloading* was what I'd had for lunch! I'd excused myself from him for a moment and went running to my bathroom to throw up!

I now know that week one must be spent "hugging the couch," as they predicted at Roswell. So you probably won't hear from me until next weekend. You saw what happened when I tried to write an update with my chemo-brain: I wrote two, a day apart, saying almost the *same thing!* And none of you said a thing to me. You are too kind!

Another side effect, about which my book warns everyone, is "shopaholism". Luckily I have not overspent money on anything that we didn't need! Now here's where the beauty of email comes in: you can either read on about our new hot water heater or you can skip it! No eyes glazing over, no walking away — I'll never know!

It turned out that our water tank had a defective part, so I was not imagining it when I thought we should have had more hot water! My plumber did not think we should put money into a ten-year-old tank; and even though I was well aware that he wanted to make a sale, I also agreed with him and convinced Warren to buy a new one. We're all happier. In this muddy season, I can hose the dogs, and shower myself without running out of hot water!

Apparently, shopaholism manifests itself in other ways as well. I read that there are a high percentage of breast cancer patients who remodel their kitchens. I guess it's a sense of control or some form of the "*I deserve this*" mentality.

While I like my kitchen, I did have another yearning a couple of weeks ago when I was feeling depressed about this long, cold winter. I told Warren that I wanted to take the dogs on a long vacation to a warm, sunny place next winter. He said, "Well, you'd better go out right now and get a job so you can start saving up!" He has always been the go-to guy for reality checks. I had to laugh at the image of me with my bald head and tiny brain applying for any job!

Before I had children, I was a teacher at the Park School of Buffalo, my alma mater. After my children were all born, I worked there part-time in the Development Office. Now I am a volunteer for them and for the Boys & Girls Clubs of Buffalo. I have had to take a leave from both while I deal with my present situation, and I appreciate the support and understanding the people at both places have provided. I am hopeful that when I return to them in the fall, I'll have a better brain and more hair above it! I also plan to volunteer at Roswell for the Patient Advocate's Office. Having been through this experience, I think I can be helpful to people there.

I have resisted the urge to order things from catalogs with two exceptions: a great new toy for the dogs, called a "Booda Wing", their favorite tug and retrieving toy, and new sheets, very smooth. Ours were all torn and semi-repaired from the days when the dogs were younger and kept having uncontrollable impulses to completely strip the bed. Too much information?

The only side effect that will stay with me until September is a constantly dripping nose. I thought it was the weather, but I just read that it's a common side effect of the Cytoxan. So I feel great, carry tissues wherever I go, and since the weather is lovely, plan to go on a nice, long walk right now.

　　We're going to Washington for the weekend, then back into La-La-Land with chemo round #3 on Monday.

　　Take care.

　　Love, Patty

Friday, April 19
4:27 P.M.

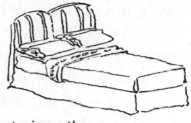

This is the third Friday I have felt this relieved to be re-entering the planet Earth! I think we are seeing a predictable pattern forming in each cycle, and I'm thrilled! What a day to come out of La-La-Land. I do remember glimpses during the week of some pretty weather through my window, and Warren was playing lots of golf; but I was sleeping most of the time and more nauseous than the other times, unfortunately. The doctor said it would be a cumulative reaction, but at least we know when we get to Friday, the worst is over!

On a day like this, it's easy to stay distracted from the queasiness! The dogs and I spent a long time at the park. It was so wonderful! I mentioned to a bald friend of mine that Warren never told me how great it feels to have a warm breeze sliding along the top of my head! He said, "Yes, but when it rains, it's really noisy!"

As I've mentioned, I'm keeping copies of all of your funny comments. I am amused by the invitations I've been receiving from some of you to go to your homes and do housework or move furniture while you're sleeping! Speaking of sleeping, let me tell you about our new sheets: they're very smooth and soft and I reeeeally appreciated them this week! I think they can be even smoother, but Warren kept bringing me food in bed, and I've been lying on crumbs for a few nights. I'll give them a good test when I'm better! And you won't ever have to know about it! Too much information! It is time to put the story of the sheets to bed!

I may be a little queasy, but it didn't stop me today from going to get a haircut. It's not that my wig is growing, but my sister told me I looked a little too much like Mrs. Doubtfire, so I asked wonderful Joe, the wig man, to cut bangs and I am 100% happier. With my mother gone, I have to rely on the honesty of friends and family, so *out with it!* We have a long road ahead of us here! One book mentioned that all cancer patients hear endless compliments about how beautiful they look. The advice is to soak it up because we'll never hear that stuff again. While that is all true, I also count on a sprinkling of honesty, please, or I'll look (and act) ridiculous!

Tuesday, I left the door open for a friend of mine because I couldn't get out of bed. She's an interior decorator and was returning a chair she had fixed. I had wanted her to see how I'd placed the furniture my brother had sent up here from my mother's apartment. Even though I was in my nauseous stupor, I am pretty sure I remember her letting herself out saying, "I can't wait to rearrange your whole living room! It's lopsided!" Apparently I hadn't gleaned enough from my Feng Shui book! Hey, I appreciated her honesty! Let's hope she's up for it at 3:00 A.M.!

Please don't be worried about me if you don't hear from me. As you can see, my life is just not that exciting! Dr. Lisa or I will be giving me the shots of Neupogen each day for a week, and I should sail through the next two weeks without incident!

Happy Spring!

Love, Patty

Monday, April 22
1:54 PM

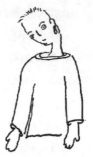

For those of you who have been wondering (and worrying) about how I always seem so upbeat, I thought today would be a perfect day to share my feelings of the moment: ***THIS SUCKS!*** I don't know whether it's because I have been nauseated all weekend or because it's April 22 and snowing. Probably none of the above, but rather because I slept only two hours last night and, as many of you already know about me, my solution for any of life's problems is a good night's sleep!

After Thursday, I tried to avoid the "amnesia" pills, but found no relief from the nausea with the bland foods that had worked in the past. Dr. Levine and his assistant, Sharon, had predicted that the effects will be cumulative and they have, in fact, been getting worse. Warren, my brother, and my friend Ellen have been urging me to take the anti-nausea meds, but I resisted because I didn't like being sooooo out of it!

Let me give you a couple of examples of how

the days went when I was on those pills: I noticed at the end of the week that we had a new storm door to the dog kennel. I have no recollection of anyone being here to install it, and **I KNOW** Warren didn't do it. There actually is a receipt with my signature on it!

On another day, I do remember being hot and wishing we had our screens in the windows. I do not remember a conversation with my window cleaner, either Tuesday or Wednesday, but I must have used the "cancer card" because all of our screens were in and the windows were cleaned, both insides and outsides, by Thursday. Now you have to understand that I have *no memory* of him and his son being here, not even when they were doing the four windows in my bedroom while I was in bed! My calculations put Ray in my bedroom for at least a half an hour! I remember none of it. He is very trustworthy, has been with us ever since we were married, did my mother-in-law's windows even before that, and is a good friend — for all I know, he's an even better friend now! (Okay, erase that image!) So do you see why I wanted my brain back?

I did finally give in and took the pills on

Saturday midnight and slept until 8:00 A.M., which was great. But I have a headache now, which I used to experience maybe once a decade! Believe me, taking Tylenol used to be a big deal for me. I liked being in control and happy all by myself. I've been taking turns feeling scared that the doctors might not know what they're doing and angry that they know *exactly* what they're doing and my body is paying the price!

Kambel is moaning. I think I've made *him* depressed. I'll bundle up and take him for a walk. Oh there, I feel much better now that I've had this self-pity session.

Thanks for letting me unload.

Love, Patty

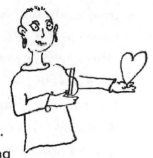

There is no substitute for a good night's sleep, and I just came out of one. I feel great. Thank you all so much for being my sounding board. I hope there won't be too many updates with the low tone of the last one, but you are my support group and I appreciate it. Remember, the beauty of email is you don't have to actually read these. You can delete them out-of-hand, or scroll down to the facts you care about, or be honest with me and tell me it's too much information and I ramble, or correct my grammar and/or spelling (I love that, really). You are *not* going to be tested on this stuff! If you're too afraid or too polite to be honest, when you see me or want to write back, you can pretend you read them and all you have to say is that you're glad I feel great! You'd be right on!

Warren walked in at the end of that day when I was feeling down and I asked him if he'd received my last email. He said, "YES, that was the worst one yet!" He thinks they're way too long, with way too much information that no one cares about, and I ramble. I wonder if I were writing about golf if he'd enjoy them.

Speaking of golf, I hope you read Tom Friedman's column in the Sunday *New York Times*. He is the most knowledgeable person, in the opinion of most people, on the Mid-East; his piece on Sunday criticized the coverage of events in the Mid-East by the major news networks. The title of the article was "Why the Golf Channel Is the Best Channel on TV."

Please understand, he (Warren, not Tom Friedman) is there for me in every possible way I want, but you'll notice he is *deleted* from the update list! My mother would agree with him 100%, not wanting ever to burden anyone with her problems. We've always been a "cry in the shower" group here. I admit, these writing sessions are actually very selfish and great help for me.

Having said that, here we go... I feel good. I am feeling slight back pain which must be my bone marrow expanding a little more from the Neupogen. But it's not even close to the first time I had this, so I don't have to stand up to keep typing. Luckily, I am very short and can reach the keys easily if it comes to that! The queasy feeling is minor, and the feeling of air pockets behind my eyes seems gone. This is different from "the air between my ears" problem, which describes my mental capacity!

Other than Warren's immediate negative response to my last email that day, he was in a *very* agreeable mood when he walked in. I had all the material about the Park School Capital Campaign spread out on the counter, ready for a long discussion about how much we should give. It took him ten seconds to agree with my suggestion and I was speechless!

Do you think it was because I'd had such a tough weekend and he felt sorry for me? Or do you think he knows how much I owe to Park for my happy, enthusiastic nature and self-confidence? Or could it be, after 9/11, he feels the nostalgia so many of us feel and wants me to give something back and help make the world a better place? Park School taught me how to write, but we *know* what he thinks of that!

Or...do you think it was because it was the day after the Drew Bledsoe trade and he wanted me completely silent so he could read the paper and be able to hear everything that everyone on TV was saying?! This is very exciting for the Buffalo Bills and for the whole city! Press conference today! And I feel good.

I feel good enough to be able to go to a funeral today. Our friend had a brain tumor and put up a dignified struggle for years. Whenever we saw her, she had on her turban and a big smile! She was another one of my inspirations. Her mother has now watched two of her children die. Our challenges are very small in comparison.

Tonight we'll be going to the University of Buffalo. I've had tickets to the Distinguished Speaker Series for a few years, and I've always gone with a friend. Tonight Ken Burns is speaking and Warren wants to go. I certainly agree — that's someone worth hearing!

Have a great day!

Love, Patty

I feel so wonderful that I am looking forward to ironing as soon as I finish this update. The last week became better as I discovered the foods that are to become my new best friends: potatoes, peanut butter, pretzels, popcorn, poached eggs, poultry, purified water, pancakes, and pop (actually, ginger ale, but I'm enjoying the alliteration).

I've eaten more potatoes in the last three months than I've eaten in the last three decades! I used to think they were empty calories, opting for empty calorie selections in the form of chocolate, but I have come to appreciate the potassium in a potato and, of course, its soothing effect on my stomach. I made a big bowl of mashed Yukon Golds this week, using skim milk and Benecol, instead of butter.

Lisa had brought the Benecol over here for Warren to help him rethink his eating habits and lower his extremely high cholesterol. He has refused to touch it, not being a substitution type guy. You should have seen his face last summer each time Susan cooked up some vegetables and tofu and tried to convince him to try *that*!

All my cancer books warn people going into chemo to avoid their favorite foods because they will associate the nausea with those foods. That has come to pass. Blueberries, broccoli, and even chocolate make me gag! I told Sharon that I was experiencing longer periods of nausea and she suggested that I go back on the three days of steroids. That will be worth a try if they make the difference.

I also mentioned to her that I was feeling light-headed and had several episodes of heart palpitations. Since I had read that one percent of people on Adriamycin have heart problems, I hoped I wasn't one of them. She assured me that the symptom of congestive heart failure, of which I should be aware, is a feeling of my legs getting thick. That struck me funny and I got her laughing with me as I said that my legs *look* thick, but what a relief that they don't *feel* thick!

Speaking of expanding, my bone marrow was doing its expanding a couple of times, but at least now I know to take Motrin and the throbbing doesn't scare me because I know what's going on in there. I feel confident the Neupogen is stimulating my white blood cells and helping me sail through days #10 through #14 without infection. Oh dear, let's say "*breeze through*" instead of "*sail* through." No more boating metaphors: I am just starting to feel like I've come off a long, rocky voyage at sea. But ahoy, land is in sight and I expect to have a terrific week ahead.

I hope the same for you!

Love, Patty

Thursday, May 2
5:54 A.M.

It's 5:30 AM and since I can't sleep, I thought I'd talk to all of you! Isn't email wonderful? I don't have much to say, so maybe this one won't be as long as those other long ones about which I heard negative comments. Warren's off the list again. One of our friends forwarded to him the one when he was deleted and he liked it, so I put him back on; but when I handed him the last one to read, he gave it right back to me after reading only a few lines. He said, "*I just don't want to read about mashed potatoes!*"

For a while I thought it was a gender issue, until I heard a negative comment from a female as well. I loved the rest of your responses. Thank you for the recipes for potato dishes! I also received a book on the Great Irish Famine. It's about how the potato blight destroyed the "important and essential potato crop, the Irish people's main source of food."

Let me quickly say here that I am not going

ahead with a complete book report! But I have nothing else to report this time (a la Seinfeld) so this will be shorter.

I do want to put everyone on notice: when you see me, do not hug me. Hugs shift my wig. One elderly friend greeted me by grabbing my neck last week and almost sent my wig into orbit! I often feel like Abe Lincoln anyway. Remember that Johnny Carson skit when he came on stage as Abe Lincoln wearing his top hat, then took off the hat and the hair was just as high? That's how I feel. May I suggest a friendly smile, a hearty, firm handshake, or a French kiss —one kiss on each cheek (not lips and tongue!). One friend told me the French greeting is three kisses instead of two, but I think we'd get dizzy!

We had Lisa's birthday party here last night and it was fun to see all of her friends. Sarah and she took care of everything, so all I had to do was buy some tulips and gerbera daisies. What a lift! Now's a good time to move all the chairs back into place. You know how I like to move furniture when I can't sleep!

Au revoir, Patty

Friday, May 10
12:09 PM

I am happy to be emerging from my troublesome week with few complaints. The pills kept me out of it and sleeping and I am feeling much better this morning.

I wish I could say the same for poor Kambel, the Golden Retriever. His stomach is in much worse shape than mine, thanks to Warren! They went to watch a Nichols softball game on Wednesday, and Warren gave Kambel a golf ball to play with. Kambel swallowed it and the emergency vet said it should be removed. Dr. Brown performed golf ball excision yesterday and took out some other inappropriate objects as well! Kambel will be coming home in a couple of hours and will have to fast for a while, then join me on a bland diet for a few days.

For me, the halfway point has been reached! Sharon described the next drug and its side effects as very different. Taxol is a plant product and the doctors have to premedicate me with steroids the day before I take it in order to prevent an anaphylactic reaction. They'll give me an IV of Benadryl and Pepcid for one hour, then a three-hour drip of the Taxol.

The good news is that the nausea will be less of a concern, but the possible bad news is that I'll be feeling tingling and numbness in my fingers and toes. Let's hope those effects are minimal since my life is walking dogs and writing to all of you! I need fingers and toes!

I could start singing, but last week when I was in a great mood, I started singing an Ella Fitzgerald favorite and Warren told me to *keep it down!* I saw that he had found a good Perry Mason rerun on TV, but my advice to anyone who happens to find a cancer patient singing: let him or her *sing!* He's probably jealous because during Chapel at Nichols, they told him to mouth the words! (PS, at Park School everyone sang!) So let's all sing together, "Oh what a beautiful morning!"

Love, Patty

Tuesday, May 14
4:32 AM

I have gas.

Be careful what you ask for, all of you with the good-natured complaints. You asked for just the facts. So instead of fluff about potatoes (and I do make fluffy potatoes!) I thought I'd hit you with the fact that I have gas. This is different from being full of hot air or being long-winded. I've improved from being nauseated to having a chronic stomachache and slight acid reflux, which woke me up, so you're going to hear all about it!

This should pass (as they say) soon, and both Kambel and I will feel better each day. Warren brought Kambel home with a baggie containing all the things the vet found in his stomach: a black chewed piece of a hockey puck, a part of a stuffed animal, and a golf ball size hunk of rawhide. There was no golf ball after all. That might be one of the few golf balls that Warren has lost. He has forever been known for being able to follow his and everyone else's in his foursome — rough, trees, water — not a problem. In Florida once, he found our friend's ball wedged into a really ripe grapefruit! He noticed the dripping from the tree. I was just along for the walk and was pretty excited about plucking grapefruits for everyone to eat!

But enough about golf; let's talk about Arnold Palmer. He said his Rottweiler once swallowed *four* (golf balls, not grapefruits). So Warren still has a long way to go to match Arnold, his idle [sic] for sure.

My stomachache might be a result of over-eating. Last night, Lisa's boyfriend, Greg, had a dinner for Sarah's birthday (28) at his house and Lisa suggested that Warren and I surprise her by being there too. Since Sarah *hates* surprises, Lisa also suggested I show up with Sarah's favorite — you guessed it, mashed potatoes. It was so much fun! Greg, Lisa, Sarah's boyfriend Tim, and Sarah's roommate Nora made everything delicious. I had been really excited about it all day, not only because birthdays are a *really* big deal in our family, but also because I don't get out much! (My choice – please, no pity here!)

Nora does hair and makeup at Papillon, a salon on Delaware Avenue, and she's going with me to the American Cancer Society's class, "Look Good, Feel Better," where we'll learn how to put makeup on a cancer face. Nora wants to learn that technique for her current and future clients going through this. My brows and lashes are almost all gone now, but I couldn't schedule a class until June 10, so I'll have to "Look Bad, Feel Worse" until then. I am kidding. I actually feel better. I burped.

Boy, is it a good thing Warren's deleted from the list. He'd kill me for all this babble! Somewhere in the course of conversation at dinner last night, Warren signed up with Nora as her newest client! Not for makeup, but it turns out he's been looking for a new person to cut his hair! So a good time was had by all.

Speaking of haircuts, the vet shaved the bottom parts of Kambel's front legs for the IV's. The poor dog looks like he's wearing kneesocks!

Hope you all feel as good as *you* look!

Good night.

Love, Patty

Tuesday, May 14
10:17 AM

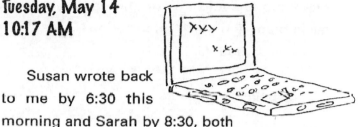

Susan wrote back to me by 6:30 this morning and Sarah by 8:30, both of them pointing out the mistake: Arnold Palmer is not Warren's idle but rather his idol! (Lisa doesn't bother to read them when they're long.) Susan's line made my day: "Didn't bother to proof-read, huh?" (Of course I make mistakes even when I do proof read!) Hey, is that two words or one?

I am happy to provide my children with the satisfaction of catching a parent in the act of doing something wrong that the parent has been harping on for a *lifetime*! They all rejoiced when Warren had his New York Thruway EZPass suspended for a month because he went through a lane too fast!

I could try to blame the gas, but another thing they always hear me say is: "OFFER NO EXCUSES!"

I feel much better after a couple of hours of

sleep and a giant bowl of shredded wheat and raisin bran! Too much information?

Have a good day!

Love, Patty

Wednesday, May 29
7:08 P.M.

I feel maaahvelous! Warren
dropped me off at Roswell
yesterday at 8:30 AM and my friend
Devon met me there and
entertained me until we
walked out at 4:00 PM. The
time really did go fast. First I had my blood
drawn, then met Sharon who explained what is
going to happen to me for the next four chemo
sessions.

Here it is: I am now on Taxol, a plant product
that will cause me to go into anaphylactic shock
(an allergic reaction) if I don't load up on pre-
medications. So I took ten Dexamethasone pills
(steroids) throughout the day before my
treatment, and the first hour in the chemo lab I
had an IV of Benadryl and Pepcid, then three
hours of the Taxol.

I did feel queasy the whole time I was there
and the nurse said that I was experiencing
"anticipatory nausea," a common response to all
the nausea associated with the last chemo

"cocktail". Devon happened upon some herbal tea with camomile, which helped my stomach. As soon as I walked into my house, I felt wonderful, like stepping off a rocky boat! The good news is that Taxol will not cause nausea, nor will it cause my white cell count to go down, so I don't have to give myself any more Neupogen shots.

I have had so much energy today, which Lisa says is from the steroids. I think it's also because it has been a beautiful day and I have to take advantage of the good weather and my state of well-being! I hauled a bookshelf up from the basement, cleaned the garage, carried the clay pots out to the patio, walked Kambel for an hour, ran errands and was on such a roll that I went out twice without remembering my wig! One reason I was scurrying around is the reported side effect of Taxol on days #3 through #6: my doctors predict that I will feel like I have been hit by a truck, my body will ache all over, but that will go away by day #7! Motrin will help and *nothing* will be as bad as nausea!

So I *am happy*! The tingly and numb fingers and feet won't develop until a few more doses and they will slowly feel better through September. My hair will start to grow now, but only one inch. Then it will stop until the Taxol is done, so I'll have a one-inch brush cut! Sharon thought one inch was no big deal, but I assured her that one inch on a short person is *significant*. I have lied about that inch for years! I am also chubby. I've gained ten pounds and can't seem to stop craving those potatoes! I believe a bald head looks better with cheek bones, but I will never let vanity get in the way of this euphoria!

Be well.

Love, Patty

Monday, June 3
12:54 P.M.

I feel so good that I am wondering if they forgot to put the Taxol in my drip! The warmer weather has felt great, too. I've been walking around the neighborhood with the dogs and without my hair. Not only does it feel more comfortable, but also I am convinced that sunshine will help my hair grow! It works for grass!

One pleasing side effect of the last drug was the loss of my facial hair. Let's hope that the inch, which Sharon promised, does not grow in as a mustache instead of a brush cut!

Another reason I don't wear the wig most of the time is because it's hot! It washes easily, but I have to be careful where I hang it to dry. I found Kambel running through the house with it, so excited. I really couldn't blame him — when it hangs on a doorknob or lies on a counter it looks like a squirrel!

Enjoy yourselves and feel as good as I do!

Love, Patty

Monday, June 17
6:05 P.M.

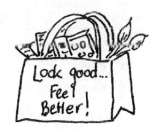

I think a pattern is forming where the better I feel, the less I write! The session today went smoothly. Warren dropped me off at 8:00 and I was home by 4:00. My friend Trudy met me there and helped make the time fly.

Dr. Levine wanted to talk to me because he hadn't seen me in a long time. I was able to ask him if he was sure the lab put any Taxol in the drip last time because I had *no* side effects. He said that while that was rare, I should feel lucky and not worry! He said I should be prepared for the truck to hit me on days #3 through #6 of this week, because the effects are cumulative, and I may not be lucky again. If that's the case ... I'll take Motrin and be fine!

Nora went with me to the American Cancer Society's "Look Good, Feel Better" class last week where we received a big bag of free makeup! (Remember Nora is Sarah's roommate and Warren's new hairdresser.) She did a masterful job on my eyebrows and taught me. My purpose for going was accomplished and we left early.

My next chemo sessions are July 8 and July 29. Then I'll be finished. I'll have radiation during the last two weeks of August, going every day until the end of September. Then I'll take Arimidex for five years and be watched closely. Arimidex is an estrogen antagonist, like Tamoxifen but with fewer problematic side effects. It blocks the body's use of estrogen, attacking the estrogen receptors in whatever cancer cells might try to grow.

Time is flying.

Enjoy yourselves.

Love, Patty

Sunday, June 23
6:32 A.M.

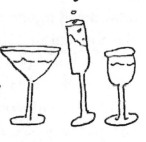

There's been a hair sighting. Lisa walked in the other day and exclaimed, "You have hair!" We've had painters here for weeks, sanding and scraping, and she found me cleaning and dusting, so I was inclined to believe it was merely the dust settling on my head. Upon closer inspection, and with the new magnifying mirror with a bright light, which a friend gave me to help me find and draw my eyebrows, I can see peach fuzz. The better news is: no new peach fuzz on my mustache or beard!

Speaking of peaches, we were at a family Bat Mitzvah party last night and I was drinking peach champagne, yum. Lisa and Sarah wanted to cut me off, claiming I was getting loud. I had been unable to drink wine since associating it with the nausea, and I was having difficulty reintroducing myself to it, so I stuck to cosmos last week at the Cherry Hill dinner dance to be safe. Unfortunately, after three cosmos I was smashed. (It was really only two cosmos and the third down my dress; those martini glasses are way too difficult to hold up straight!)

The good news is that yesterday, after a good walk, while Warren and the girls were playing golf, my friend Michelle and I celebrated her birthday on my patio with a bottle of Sancerre, and it went down easily with no suggestion of nausea! Warren joined us (with a Snapple) and reported that he and the girls had had fun. That news coupled with the gentle breeze and the smell of the heliotrope, made life perfect. There really is nothing better than everyone in one's family being happy all at the same time!

I was supposed to feel like I had the flu without a fever, but the only feverish thing I feel is the pace I'm setting to clean the house and have it ready for a shower I'm hosting with two other friends this week. It will be fun to see many old friends. I don't even feel aches from hauling clay pots.

The "Taxol Train" took a different track!

Take care.

Love, Patty

Monday, July 8
7:58 A.M.

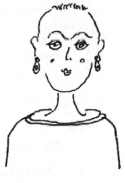

My head looks like a Ch-Ch-Ch-Chia Pet; mine's white instead of green.

I've been up since 4:00 A.M., waiting to take my last five steroids before my chemo later this morning. I puttered around the house, moved Lisa's microwave into the garage (she's moving), loaded Warren's lawnmower into the car for Sarah's friend (with Warren's help), watered flowers, and decided to send an update. I have the time but very little to say (relative to other people who don't talk too much).

Just wanted you to know I feel wonderful. My biggest problem is finding and drawing my eyebrows so they match! I often go back and forth, trying to make them even, until they almost meet in the middle! My dripping nose has stopped and all systems are go! If I do feel aches this week, it may be a result of lifting the mower and the microwave rather than from being hit by the "Taxol Train."

I am hoping the nurses take me on time today, not only because I'd like to get my friend Devon home at a reasonable hour, but also because Warren's leaving Kambel in his office when he goes to play golf. Kambel loves to shred any paper he finds on the floor, and if you've ever seen Warren's office you know why this is a concern! One time he shredded some mail before Warren had a chance to read it; one of the "chads" had the return address of the Bar Association, so that was no great loss. I reminded him of this as they were leaving this morning, but we know he does not always listen to me. Maybe I'll put him back on the update list and hope he doesn't delete this message before reading it!

It's summertime and the livin' is easy!

Enjoy it and ch-ch-ch-cheers!

Love, Patty

Tuesday, July 9
7:45 A.M.

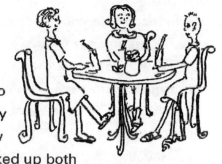

We had so much fun yesterday that the time flew by. They were backed up both in the Breast Clinic, where I saw Dr. Levine, and in the chemo lab, where they had ninety patients scheduled and only eight nurses. But after waiting an hour, Devon and I took a beeper and went to lunch in the cafeteria.

I called my new best friend, the Patient Advocate, who had helped me in the hospital. She had told me to be sure to call her if I ran into any problems, so I left a message for her from the patient lounge, and by the time we walked back to the chemo lab, she was there waiting for us!

She knew I had four hours of chemo ahead of me and she arranged for me to be taken immediately; she said she was going to stay around to make sure my orders came down so they could start me in a timely manner. (I have been experiencing another one-hour wait once I am placed in a chair in the lab. The long waits are sometimes inevitable in any chemo lab anywhere, so I encourage anyone who has to go through this to seek out and take advantage of the services of a patient advocate if one is available.)

Having read my email in the morning, our friend Mary Ellen surprised us with a visit and offered to rescue Kambel from Warren. She had lunch with us, then took Kambel to play with Henry, her chocolate Lab, all afternoon! We picked him up by 5:30 and I was home by 6:00. The time really did fly as Devon and I discussed and solved most of the world's problems.

I told Dr. Levine earlier that he should feel as good as I feel, and he laughed, saying that my reaction has been quite unusual and I should feel lucky and enjoy it. I assured him that I'm thrilled but had to ask again if he was sure he had given me enough of the poison. He read my chart and felt confident.

He asked me to choose a radiologist, and, all of them being equal, I picked the one closest to my home because I'll be going every day for six or eight weeks, starting in mid-August. So, Dr.

Levine will send my file over to Dr. O'Connor, at Buffalo Medical Group, and arrange my first appointment with him in a few weeks to set things up.

We're really moving along! As we progress closer to the time when I will start the hormonal therapy for five years, he wants to discuss the pros and cons of Arimidex vs. Tamoxifen. Arimidex is a new drug and I have been reading that it is controversial. He agreed and said it will be a long discussion; Lisa wants to be in on that and I'll keep you posted.

I hope all is going well for you.

Love, Patty

Tuesday, July 30
5:52 A.M.

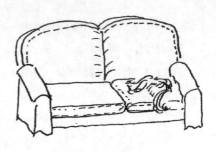

The last treatment was the easiest and fastest. My suggestion to anyone going through these is to try to book early appointments! Blood work was at 8:00 A.M. and I saw Dr. Levine at 8:30. Warren, Lisa, Trudy, and I all listened to the pros and cons of Tamoxifen versus Arimidex. In summary, they both work by exerting an effect on estrogen, which feeds my cancer and helps it grow. A five-year study is showing Arimidex to be more effective. Arimidex limits the amount of estrogen the body produces, while Tamoxifen blocks estrogen from binding to the cancer receptors in the breast. Both drugs cause hot flashes, but unlike Tamoxifen, Arimidex does not cause blood clots or increase the risk of uterine cancer. (Early studies show this for 1/2 of 1% of the 9,000 women tested.)

The down side to being on Arimidex: women taking this drug have more problems with bone thinning and fractures. Tamoxifen blocks estrogen in the breast, but it acts like a weak estrogen outside the breast, so it stimulates bone and keeps it from getting thin. Arimidex, on the other hand, works by preventing the production of estrogen. Since I already have osteopenia (the precondition for osteoporosis), Arimidex may not be the right choice for me. Even though I am taking Fosomax, to strengthen by bones, Dr. Levine admitted that it might not be strong enough to counter the effects of the Arimidex.

We have several weeks to weigh the pros and cons because I won't start hormone therapy until after radiation, which I hope will start August 19 and go through October 11. By then we'll make a decision. Lisa and I are leaning towards Tamoxifon because of the bone issue; Warren likes the statistics with Arimidex improving overall survival rates. As more study results become available, Dr. Levine expects that over another five to ten years, we'll see a greater difference between the effectiveness of the two drugs and fewer recurrences in distant organs among women taking Arimidex.

We've been having a wonderful summer,

with out-of-town friends coming to visit over the last two weekends and many activities as we take advantage of the beautiful weather! One day last week, I was ready with our bags packed on the counter when Warren picked us up and we headed for Canada. Warren was going to be playing golf, while Kambel and I would be playing on the beach with friends. We planned to meet for dinner at Lucy's, a great restaurant in Port Colborne.

As we approached the Peace Bridge, I reached in the bag behind my seat for my wig. NO WIG. I tore through the bag, even though I knew I had put the wig on top. I felt under Kambel — no luck. I thought it might have fallen out on the driveway or perhaps Kambel had taken it out of my bag before we left and shredded it to pieces! I had visions of never going to a social function until February! We called our friend and neighbor Michelle who ran over to the house and called us back to report no hair sighting on the driveway. I asked her to check Kambel's favorite stashing spot on a couch, and *there* it was, and intact! I was feeling both relief and trepidation. The thought of going to a restaurant with a bald head scared me.

I said to Warren, "This is a real test of character!"

Clueless, he asked, "Whose? Yours or Kambel's?"

Honestly, his reaction and that of my friends made it easier for me. Since Lucy's, I've been going more places with just my fuzzy head and feeling cooler and more comfortable. I believe that as long as I smile at the people who stare at me, it assures them that I'm feeling great and then they feel comfortable too.

Stay cool yourselves!

Love, Patty

Wednesday, July 31
7:55 P.M.

I want to record my
first tingly toes, fingers,
and feet today; the only
record I have is in my
updates, and anyway ... I
thought you'd want to
know! Frankly, I was
relieved, once I realized
what was happening,
because it appears
that the Taxol is doing what was predicted. The
sensation is ever so slight and not bothersome.

After the last email about Kambel taking my
wig, my sister replied, *"Dear God, give me
strength. When are you going to put safeguards
in place that insure that creature does not get his
slimy mouth all over your stunning hair?! I
suppose it doesn't matter because I'm sure your
little pinhead looks cute with your green eyes.
Mom would remind you to always wear
earrings! Love, Cathy."*

My brother was in town on business today
and came over for a quick bite to eat before

driving back to Ann Arbor. He hadn't seen me since my hair fell out. At the first sight of me, he doubled over, convulsed in laughter, then hugged me and wouldn't stop rubbing my head. He had read my last email and pointed to my head, saying, "So your dog took your wig and you actually went out in public like that?" *A sense of humor is a sense of proportion* (Dag Hammarskjold).

I assured him that Kambel did me a huge favor; now in this heat I go everywhere without it! One day last week I was a little disappointed when I ran into a person who mistook me for someone's mother. When I confessed my vanity to Warren, he didn't get it. He said, "Well, you ARE someone's mother." I explained that the *someone* was forty years old.

My brother and I had a fast but good visit and he was on his way, armed with all kinds of questions he wants to ask his doctor-friends about my treatment decisions.

I'm welcoming as many opinions as there are out there. I'm still leaning towards the Tamoxifen so that my bones don't start "leaning" from the Arimidex!

Speaking of my bones, I have asked a friend of mine who teaches at the University of Buffalo Medical School to do me a favor. Before my cancer diagnosis, I had the back of my driver's license filled out for organ donation. Now that my parts are no longer valuable for that, I thought I'd make myself useful as a cadaver. I asked my friend for the name of the person I should call at the Med School to arrange for my body to be sent there when I die.

I assured him that I am not expecting to die soon, but I wanted to have all the paperwork done well before I die. Whenever he felt inclined to deal with this matter was fine with me. There was no rush.

His response: *"Glad you are not planning this soon. I will scope it out for you with the department of anatomy and let you know at my leisure over the next millennium."*

Meanwhile, let's enjoy this splendid weather!

Love, Patty

Thursday, August 1
5:41 P.M.

My ear is throbbing. Unrelated to the chemo, it has had a mysterious growth on the top that would not heal. It had been hurting for a few months, especially when I slept on it. So, I thought it was time to have it seen by a doctor. He carved it off today, stitched it up and told me to come back in a week to find out the results of the biopsy.

Dr. Levine had inspected it on Monday, and while he was suggesting I see someone about it, as I was lying on his table, I heard Dr. Lisa, deeply concerned, standing at my feet saying, "Someone needs a pedicure!"

It's time to be on my patio, enjoying every last breezy evening of summer, and instead of Tylenol, I am choosing Sancerre!

Love, Vincent Van Gogh

Thursday, August 8
8:05 PM

My doctor took out the five stitches from my ear today and informed me that the patholo-gy report reveals *hyperkeratosis, chondrodermatitis nodularis helicis*. In other words, I'm fine!

The cold, numb, and tingly sensation in my hands is mild and infrequent. My feet feel good (and look good after the pedicure)!

Feel good yourselves!

Love, Patty

Monday, August 19
9:18 P.M.

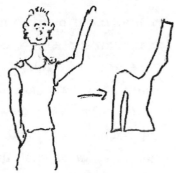

Warren and I met Dr.
O'Connor in his offices
at the Buffalo Medical
Group on Essjay Road
last Wednesday. He examined me, read my case
history, and explained the plan he had in mind
for me. I will be going every weekday, starting
tomorrow, for thirty-six treatments. Each one will
take no more than a couple of minutes, so I will
be in and out of there in approximately ten
minutes each day, feeling nothing.

The standard number of times for radiation
therapy is twenty-eight on the entire breast area;
then he'll be "boosting the resection site" (the
site of my tumor) with eight additional
treatments, concentrating on that smaller area.
He made that determination based on my life
expectancy. I like his thinking!

I went back Friday and his assistant made a
mold of my body (waist up), with my arm up
over my head, by laying me on a plastic bag
filled with gooey stuff which hardened. I will lie

in that mold every time to keep myself in the exact same position. She took two x-rays, one front and one side, for the doctor to see the treatment area. I also had a CT scan.

The size of the treatment area, the angle of the machine, and the distance of the machine are the parameters that the doctor will transpose onto the CT scan image of my breast. His objective is to angle the radiation in such a way as to maximize the amount of rays to the whole breast, while minimizing the amount to my lung. Hmm. They drew purple marks and gave me one tattoo, marking the spot for them to see where to zap me.

My instruction sheet says to avoid long, hot showers (refer back to the updates about the new hot water tank) for six to nine months, until my skin is back to normal! Let's hope for a warm fall — you know how I love to shower for an hour! Speaking of showers, I am taking a survey among all my bald friends to find out how to wash a bald head while my hair starts to grow. Should I use soap or shampoo? I've been intending to ask that for months, but I always think of it in the shower where I don't have any place to write it down!

Today was my last visit to Roswell for a few months. Sharon told me the neuropathy (tingly fingers and feet) will start to feel better through September. I asked her when I should expect my hair to start growing again. It has grown an inch and stopped. The answer: TODAY! It has been three weeks since the Taxol treatment, so I am chemo-free. I stood out in the rain today, hoping that might speed things along.

One observation today: As I was looking for a parking place in the Roswell ramp, I saw a man about to pull into an available spot; then he saw me and stopped, motioning for me to take it instead. At first I was surprised and waved a thank you. But as I was walking away, I realized that he'd noticed my bald head and felt sorry for me, as he saw a cancer victim. It made me sad. I am sure in the past I had pity on my face when I saw people who looked as I look now, but I am ready as I go forward to be positive and forthright with greetings and questions. I love it when strangers do that to me!

Stay well.

Love, Patty

Monday, August 26
5:34 P.M.

No news is good news from me. The radiation has been fast and easy. I go every weekday at 10:15 and the staff is usually waiting for *me*. I'm out of there in ten minutes. They tell me to breathe normally, but I find myself holding my breath. I'll work on that! I keep thinking that if I don't breathe and keep really still, they'll be sure to get the rays in the right place!

The doctor will talk to me every Monday to make sure my skin is okay and answer any questions. Today I asked him how he determined the dose of radiation and he explained that there is only one accepted dose for breast cancer. I found that reassuring. My other question was about my tattoo: I noticed a freckle one inch below the tattoo and was worried over the weekend that the nurses were lining up with the wrong dot! I asked them how they could tell the difference and they said it was easy because one was blue!

I appreciated many of your comments after

my Roswell parking place story. One friend made me laugh with his response: *We don't feel sorry for you. We are nice to you because we like you. That guy probably saw a better parking spot!*

Speaking of Roswell, I have spoken to their Development Director about turning all these updates into some sort of publication that could be not only helpful and/or entertaining for others going through this, but also effective as a vehicle for fund-raising, with all the royalties going to Roswell. If this idea gets off the ground, I'll need a title. So I'm entertaining suggestions from all of you. My best idea: *Humor After The Tumor!*

Stay well.

Love, Patty

Sunday, September 8
11:38 P.M.

I don't know if I have "writer's block" or simply nothing noteworthy to write. I'll let *you* be the judge!

Right now I'm having difficulty breathing because the Bills made me want to eat! When they play poorly, Warren shakes his foot. I eat. I feel like I'm going to explode! However, I'm sure my self-control will reappear. I need to feel in control of *something*, because I don't feel in control of the cancer.

People keep suggesting to me that it must feel great to be almost done with my treatments. Actually, I feel quite the opposite. I anticipate it feeling like something of a let down. Up to now, I have been not only closely monitored by teams of doctors, but also feeling proactive in the attack! After next month, I think I'll feel more helpless. As happy as I am to notice my eyebrows growing back, they are a clear indication that all that poison is out of my body and not killing cancer cells anymore!

But enough doom and gloom. Let me tell you more about my hair: I have a white layer on my head that's been there for almost a month and growing, *plus* a visible darker undercoat that has appeared in the last week. I had a wonderful long night of sleep with a dream that my hair grew everywhere, including on my ears, unfortunately, and everyone kept telling me that I looked like a Golden Retriever. Not difficult to analyze that one since I've had major issues with hair, ear, and dog!

Speaking of Kambel, these dating services out there could tell their clients one tip: just shave your head and go everywhere with a Golden Retriever. People will want to meet you, ask all about you, the dog, and the cancer, and you can learn their life stories as well! I believe it *must* be a Golden Retriever — Ellen and I were dining on the patio at a friend's winery near St. Catharines, Ontario, but nobody gave her Miniature Poodle the time of day! (I may have just ended a beautiful forty-year friendship with that line!) Did I mention how maahvelous Ellen looks with her new short hair cut? She was the third friend to cut her hair very short after being inspired by my bald head!

The book idea seems to be taking on a life of its own, and while I appreciate everyone's enthusiasm, I must prepare all of you for the reality that no one else may be interested in it before you become too disappointed. I have one friend trying to decide who in Hollywood should play Patty in the movie!

I continue to feel slightly tingly intermittently; I'm not sure if it's from the Taxol or Warren. What do you think?

Let's hope next week is a good week for you and the Bills!

Love, Patty

Thursday, September 26
5:36 P.M.

La Shona Tova! Happy New Year in Hebrew!

It has been so long since my last update that my hair is long, compared to last month! I go *almost* everywhere without my wig now. The girls encourage it, but Warren's worried I might scare someone. I started out with it the other night at a restaurant, but it was very hot, so I peeled it off without warning and one old friend burst into tears. I assured her that I was fine.

I was tempted to go to Temple without it, but decided against that when I thought people would be in a somber enough mood and wouldn't need anything else to possibly bring them down. I figured that it was not only Yom Kippur and they'd be atoning for their sins, but also many of us were missing the Bills game and/or *The Sopranos*.

Speaking of Temple, my dermatologist is urging me to remove a mole she found on my temple. I am not worried about skin cancer, but I did ask how deep a plastic surgeon would have to drill. I can't afford any more brain tampering!

I have been experiencing severe short-term memory loss, and I've been losing and forgetting things on a regular basis. The doctor assured me that the incision will be quite superficial. I wonder if I could ask him to pull my skin up nice and tight! Of course my insurance won't cover the other side so I'd look cockeyed.

I plan to wait until I have more hair. I hope I'll soon have more on my head than on the rest of my face. While I am thrilled to once again have eyebrows and lashes, I could do without the rest of this facial hair. At this rate, I'll be wrestling Warren for the Gillette Foamy! There were many little bumps all over my body for a while which the dermatologist explained were all my hair follicles getting pumped up and ready to sprout hairs, which they have done. So now I'm smooth and furry. Too much information?

Smoothly is the word to use for how the radiation is going. I am in and out of there each day in a flash! Buffalo Medical Group is only fifteen minutes from my house, which is why I picked it. Kambel has caught on to the routine and starts to moan at me around 10:00 every morning —- he *loves* a car ride! I am starting to notice pinkness on my skin. It looks like someone was ironing me and left the iron in that one place too long, sort of a medium-rare triangle right now.

The doctor checks me every Monday, and if I start to look too raw, he'll stop the treatments until the skin improves. I'm not expecting that to happen and neither is he as I am diligent about moisturizing the area. While I lie in my body mold with my arm up behind my head each time, other women have described a different technique used at Roswell where they lie on a board and hold onto a handle. Both techniques serve the purpose of keeping us in the same position each time. I plan to take my mold home with me and invite anyone with an artistic bent to submit ideas for how to paint me!

I am having a difficult time deciding whether or not to go back to soy milk. Soy is a weak source of estrogen, and since my cancer is estrogen-driven, I wonder if I should drink it or not. Dr. O'Connor says if I like it, drink it in moderation. Dr. Lisa says that since I don't do anything in moderation, and since zero estrogen is better than some estrogen, I should nix it. Your comments and opinions are encouraged.

We're looking forward to visiting Warren's sister, Linda, in Philadelphia this weekend. It will be fun to spend time with her daughters, Leslie and Marcy, and their families.

Back to my hair (luckily there's not too much hair on my back), I am convinced that now with the winds of autumn picking up, I can feel hairs MOVE!

Enjoy the season.

Love, Patty

Wednesday, October 2
7:08 A.M.

On Monday, Dr. O'Connor and his assistants spent almost an hour taking pictures and x-rays, and looking through a flouroscope to view my excision site from the front and side. All this was in preparation for eight more sessions of what they call a "boost" to that site. Using an electronic cone, they aim the rays more directly onto the spot.

Dr. O'Connor had mentioned at the outset of all the radiation treatments that it would be easy for him to find the spot where the tumor had been because Dr. Edge had marked the area well. On Monday, when he mentioned that again, I asked him how Dr. Edge had marked the spot. He said that he left little metal clips in there! So as I was lying there yesterday, I pictured myself setting off all kinds of alarms at airport security checkpoints. I asked and was assured that these clips are the size of little staples and won't cause a problem!

The doctor said that I have tolerated the

treatments well and made him look like he knows what he is doing. Very cute sense of humor. I try not to wonder about that myself! I still occasionally feel a slight tingle in my thumbs and numbness in my feet when I wake up in the morning. I shuffle around for a while until they're ready. Dancing would be out of the question at that hour.

Warren didn't notice my eyebrows until he read the last email, but he didn't read the whole thing. That was as far as he could wade through it—way too long for him. Speaking of long (again), I had to cut my hair. It was starting to stick out over my ears. I couldn't do a thing with it! Now I look like someone from Star Trek and plan to continue cutting it there until the top grows down.

It is terrific to have close friends with a sense of humor during this time of re-entry, with hair everywhere and short-term memory loss. Ellen hadn't seen me in a month, and the first words out of her mouth were about my fuzzy face! (A best friend for forty years can say that!) Having read my emails about the short term memory loss, there are a few people responding with claims that I owe them money!

I am told, by those who have been through this, that the fog should lift in six to eight months! So keep reminding me who you are, stay well, and carry photo ID!

Love, Patty

Friday, October 4
9:56 PM

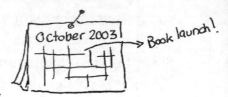

My hair is growing, my treatments are ending, re-entry into "normal" life is starting, so it's time for my updates to stop. I won't stop writing them, because they are my only record of the journey, and they will be available upon request; but this is the last one I will be sending to the entire group. And what a group you've been. Friends and family facilitated the ride and made it fast and fun! (Ya gotta love the alliteration. I guess I want to end the book with a bang!)

There *is* going to be a book. The people at Roswell are excited and encouraging as we begin what they predict will be a ten-month project. The first thing they want to do right away is to take a picture of me while I'm still semi-bald. I asked if Kambel could be in it and they said yes. There will be another picture with the whole family when only one of us is bald.

The plan is to launch it next October during Breast Cancer Awareness Month. They believe there's a niche in the marketplace for a first-person account by an "ordinary" person, someone to whom people can relate. Also, they think it has appeal because it's a group experience in an email format, and they think it's funny. I appreciate their appreciation of my sense of humor.

I want all the royalties from the sale of the book to go to Roswell, so I hope it will help people and raise money for cancer research as well. It also affords me the opportunity to stay connected to the entire experience. I'd hate to quit Cancer World cold turkey.

As I've said before, I am finding no comfort in the end of my treatments as I wonder how vigilant the doctors will be in the future. Dr. Lisa wants me to ask them how often they plan to do bone scans, x-rays, and mammograms. Meanwhile, it feels good to move off center as I busy myself with many mini-projects ahead.

I started to tell Warren all about them tonight and he started to read the paper. I told him I wasn't finished and he said, "I've heard enough." I'd say that's probably true for all of you, too.

Thanks again for being there.

Love, Patty

Wednesday, October 30
4:40 P.M.

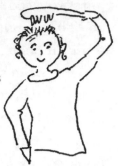

I appreciate the kind words of encouragement from many of you on my email list and I'll continue sending updates to those of you who asked to remain on the list. It's been a while since my last update because I have had very little to report; but I've been jotting little notes to myself, and the pile of little notes is growing big! While you may yawn through some or all of this, bear with me because it's my only record of things I may want to remember. My brain functions well enough to assure me that I have little memory; and there are some side effects, or minor conditions, which I think are noteworthy.

On the fourth day of the radiation "boost", there was slight blistering and more redness. Dr. O'Connor's assistant had told me I would experience the worst of the redness in one week after the last treatment. It appeared that I was right on schedule. The best thing about those thirty-six radiation sessions was the radio station piped into the room playing oldies. After listening to my favorites, I reported them to Sarah and she's burned four CD's for me so far!

Now that I am "all finished having cancer", the boost area is fading and the only effect I occasionally feel in that area is shooting pangs, like needles. The doctor said that he hears this from many women, but there is no scientific explanation for this other than the fact that the nerve endings have been "knocked around quite a bit," so they're probably going through some sort of healing process! As long as other women have reported this, I feel reassured!

I've been enjoying the vanilla rice milk every morning as a perfect substitute for the soy milk and taking walks every day with and without Kambel as I bundle up and brace myself for the long cold winter! I do have hair but not enough to keep my head warm. It is, I want you to know, enough to *brush*! I used to wonder why Warren bothered until I reached this stage myself and realized that it does look slightly more organized if large groups of hairs can move in the same direction.

Moving back to my limited brain function, I

went to a lecture on the artist Modigliani a few weeks ago and proceeded to fall sound asleep. The wine at dinner with my friends Trudy and Michelle probably didn't help! I remember that he was Jewish and had one girlfriend with a very long neck! I have seen the exhibit once and plan to go again tonight. It is *wonderful*, and I find that I retain more information when I keep walking from one masterpiece to another as I listen to an audio "wand."

I might have another problem with my brain. I woke up this morning experiencing slight dizziness. It's been better throughout the day, but every once in a while I feel like I'm going to tip over. I decided not to walk Kambel today. So I drove to the dog park instead. I know it wasn't smart to drive a car, but that's an example of my limited brain function. I'm wondering if I've cooked up this problem because I'm subconsciously disappointed that I'm "all finished having cancer." If it's not better by tomorrow I'll call Dr. Levine, but I wanted to write about it in case I forget or pass out!

The doctor did assure me that he would be monitoring me at regular intervals. I can't remember how often that will be and I didn't write that in my notebook when he said it, but I do remember feeling reassured. I'll ask him again when I see him on November 25.

HAPPY BIRTHDAY, SUSAN!   I remembered!

Love, Mommy, a.k.a Patty

Thursday, November 14
8:49 P.M.

My hair has waves developing in the back of my head and I can't stop eating the Halloween candy.

Warren walked by me as I was gnawing on a Coffee Crisp and said, "Ah, they said that drug would cause that" (referring to the Tamoxifen). If the situation gets much worse, I'll be a short, fat woman with short, fat waves. I think the best look I can hope for these days is that of a distinguished, gray haired, short *man*!

I'll just have to ride out these waves until they grow and the seasons change. People tell me that eventually one's own hair returns. In the meantime, although it looks like something you'd use to scour pots and pans, it actually feels very soft. And believe me *everyone* feels it! I don't mind; all I ask is that they put all the hairs back in the same direction when they're finished petting them.

Now that the weather is cold, I've resumed my membership at the gym. The doctors told me to put a hold on it while I was susceptible to infection, and I didn't bother to rejoin while the weather was beautiful and I could walk outside everyday with either Kambel or my friend and neighbor Michelle.

To help you picture what I look like these days, I'll tell you what happened the other morning. Michelle and I left our houses at the same time, planning to meet each other halfway. Without her glasses on, Michelle started waving at a bright blue garbage can! I didn't think about being hurt because I was laughing too hard and rationalized that at least it wasn't a fire hydrant.

I don't think that will happen again. Not because I'll be taller and slimmer, but because she is soon to have laser eye surgery.

Kambel also has kept me active. He has mastered his concept of retrieving, preferring to watch his master, me, retrieve the toys he drops far away from where I stand, while he looks on with delight!

I don't think I could ever give Kambel too much credit for helping me through this journey. Even my mother, not a dog lover herself, remarked when she was here, during the last weeks of her illness, that the dogs were comforting companions. My friend who is a veterinarian told me about studies that have proven how dogs help people cope and/or recover.

In his email about the therapeutic use of pets, he said, "*We know that just stroking a pet can reduce anxiety and lower blood pressure. Pets in the home can make an ill person feel needed. They are a distraction from worry and a source of humor and security. They stimulate and may even force physical activity.*"

Not to take anything away from Warren, but I can't see him draping himself across me as I read, or running to the door with an ecstatic greeting at the sight of me arriving home. It's taken me thirty years to persuade him to say *hello*!

Michelle is my relentless personal trainer and provides the incentive I need to go to the gym and step onto the treadmill. I have avoided the arm weights, using lymphedema as an excuse, but today I called my physical therapist at Roswell to hear a definitive answer on the subject and he gave me both good news and bad. The good news (because I'm lazy) is that he doesn't want me doing too fast a pace on the treadmill, which might put too much of a burden on the compromised lymph system! What a great excuse to cruise at a comfortable clip and let Michelle do Mach 2!

The bad news for me (because I'm lazy) is that I *can* start doing weight training again, as long as I *gradually* work up to where I was before. He explained that the rule is to avoid lifting heavy objects when my arm is *at my side*. Weight training, on the other hand (so to speak), is actually *recommended* for women after lymph node excision.

There is even a group of breast cancer survivors who row Dragon boats! In 1996, in Vancouver, B.C., Dr. Don McKenzie, a sports medicine physician and exercise physiologist, formed a team called *Abreast in a Boat*. Dr. McKenzie wanted to disprove the myth that repetitive upper body exercise in women treated for breast cancer encourages lymphedema. Dragon boating was chosen because it is strenuous, repetitive, and requires upper body strength.

His theory was proven correct.

In April 2000, western New York's Breast Cancer Survivor team was formed, calling themselves *The Hope Chest*. The team is now one of 33 international breast cancer survivor teams; they are the second team in the United States and the only breast cancer survivor team in New York State. It's inspiring information for those of you who might be motivated!

As *I* try to stay in shape, my shape has changed. Without giving too much information here, let me just say that the site where Dr. Edge cut my lump must have developed scar tissue that has cut me a new figure. You could say it's one of the "*perks*" to having the procedure! Figuratively speaking, it's another silver lining — or one more flip side to my story; but Warren would flip if I write any more about it.

You'll know, if you are reading about the shape of my breast, that Warren refused to proof-read the book for me. I'll ask one more time, and delete the above if he wants me to; but the last time I suggested that he'd be a great proof- reader, he exclaimed, "Ugh, NO! One reading was bad enough!"

I am also experiencing frequent hot flashes which are mild and welcome in what is promising to be a long, cold winter. My body's furnace is fluctuating between freezing and flashing, blending into a fine balance!

Stay well and warm.

Love, Patty

Saturday, December 7
5:00 PM

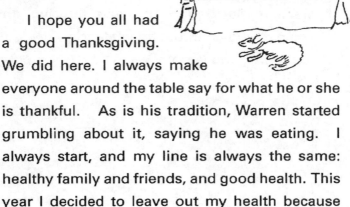

I hope you all had a good Thanksgiving. We did here. I always make everyone around the table say for what he or she is thankful. As is his tradition, Warren started grumbling about it, saying he was eating. I always start, and my line is always the same: healthy family and friends, and good health. This year I decided to leave out my health because I'm having my doubts, but everyone else mentioned that and other variations of that theme, as well as a few funny one-liners.

Even Warren rolled with the mood by the time it was his turn and said he was thankful for Patty. We were all slightly taken aback. It was a bittersweet exercise as we missed those departed and we all appreciated cousin Beverly saying that we were at least thankful for the memories of them.

I had been to Roswell earlier in that week for my three-month checkup with Dr. Levine, where I listened to answers to my long list of questions.

He will be seeing me every three months for the first two years, then every four months during the third year, every six months during the fourth year, and once a year in the fifth year and beyond. There is no reason to order a bone scan unless I have problems or pain that *won't go away*. He saw no reason to have my ovaries removed because I have no family history of ovarian cancer and I am post menopausal.

Dr. Levine wanted to know if the bottom of my feet had been numb, and I told him that I had felt the numbness when I stepped out of bed every morning through September, but now I'm fine and ready to dance.

Speaking of dancing, I asked Warren if we could spend New Year's Eve waltzing the night away with the Buffalo Philharmonic. They're presenting *A Night in Old Vienna* where Oliver's Restaurant will cater dinner and we could dance to the music of Johann Strauss, Jr. and others. I told him that I'd just purchased a new CD for my car with all of the world's favorite waltzes and they were lifting my spirits as I drove around listening to them.

Warren's response: "*Good, keep on driving*

around."

Numb feet or not, thankful or not, he's not dancing!

I am thankful for a sense of humor and for friends and family with that sense as well. I've been thinking about what a sense of humor really is. The importance of it is less about being funny and more about seeing the world in a positive way, and not taking one's self or others too seriously.

Today Lisa arranged a lunch with her friend and her friend's mother who was just diagnosed with breast cancer. She was scared and filled with all sorts of questions and we had a wonderful and emotional time. I surprised myself with my reaction to one last question she asked me. She asked me, "What advice would you give me?" My eyes welled up and I felt a lump in my throat. I really thought I was all finished being emotional, but it took me a minute to be able to speak (also because I had a huge mouthful of chicken souvlaki).

My answer to anyone will always be this: Keep your sense of humor; it's not a death sentence. Seek second opinions; and choose a medical team whose priority is your comfort, both emotional and physical. My doctors welcomed my questions and encouraged me to let them know when any side effects were problematic.

There is a helpful Breast Resource Center right in the Breast Clinic at Roswell, run by a kind person who encourages all the patients to stop in, call her, and/or email. It was a huge relief to be able to unload questions by calling her at any hour, especially in the middle of the night, when I could leave the questions in her voice mailbox then go back to sleep and hear from her when she found the answers for me! Ask if the team you're considering offers some form of guidance to help you gather information.

I'll also say, avoid toxic friends and surround yourself with happy people. Let all the upbeat, positive friends and family who want to do things for you do so, and on your terms. Enjoy all the indulgence.

Thanksgiving has come and gone, but I will never stop giving all of you thanks for helping me through what has actually been a great year. We really did have fun. You know how I love to say that life is full of trade-offs! In this case, the rewards far outweighed the regrets.

Thank you.

Love, Patty

Wednesday, December 11
1:00 PM

While I intended to end the book with the last email, I feel compelled to write one more note to all of you. Isn't there some expression about a "bad penny"? You can't get rid of me; I keep turning up! Maybe we should name the book "The History of Patty's Cancer, Part I" (a la Mel Brooks) or "The Quips That Won't Quit." You know I've always had a problem knowing when to stop talking! (Refer back to the emails about eyes glazing over, or people walking away or falling asleep.) I didn't think I could use the agreed upon title *Humor After The Tumor* if the last email left you all in tears! I do appreciate the kind and sensitive responses, especially from you men who cry! Also, I have more to say.

Today I was in Dash's Market where the produce manager, who found out about the coming book, had tears in her eyes as she asked a question. She wanted to know if the book would help people like herself who don't know what to do to help others with this illness – in her case, an elderly neighbor. I remembered feeling helpless when I was on the other side of the situation and convinced her that she should ignore the woman's requests to be left alone. I assured her that as long as she respected her friend's privacy, anything that she did, sent, or left at her door would comfort her friend. I think I've addressed this point throughout the emails, but I don't think I can overstate the overwhelming role everyone's attention played in my positive journey through Cancer World.

Another point of this email is to extend an offer to anyone else who might have questions about the cancer experience. Lisa and I can provide the opportunity for someone to hear my experiences with Lisa's medical explanations for them. I do not believe it's a good idea to impose myself on anyone, but if someone asks, Lisa and I will take our dog and pony show to whoever wants us.

Right now I'm running a *dog and Patty show*, given my lifestyle at the moment: we have *four* dogs in this house all week while Lisa and Greg are away. I have more hair on my clothes than on my head. Yet it did need trimming on the sides and back, so a friend came over Monday with scissors and yummy soup.

I ate the soup while she cut my hair, trimming the back and sides while we wait for the top to grow. I would like to point out the symmetry here: I opted to have my head shaved way back in March because people warned me that it would start to fall out in clumps "into my soup." Now here I was with my first official haircut marking the end of the whole experience, and dodging the hairs as they fell almost into my soup. Delicious!

I am losing my cheekbones as I'm gaining weight. I would like to blame the Tamoxifen, but I fear 'tis the season!

I wish you all Happy Holidays and **many** New Years filled with promise and peace.

Love, Patty

Afterword

Dr. Stephen B. Edge, M.D.,
Chair, Department of Breast and Soft
Tissue Surgery, Roswell Park Cancer Institute
Professor of Surgery, State University of
New York at Buffalo

So that's Patty's story, told as it happened. A personal and unique story. But it's also everyone's story retold with individual perspectives and personal twists by hundreds of thousands of women with breast cancer, and millions of people worldwide with cancer, every year.

Cancer is an intensely personal experience. It affects every aspect of life. Cancer can bring disfigurement, pain, suffering, and premature death. It changes a person's interaction with the world. It affects relationships with family, friends, and colleagues. Ultimately, it changes a life forever. For those who beat the disease, and even for many who don't, cancer redefines life.

Patty gives us an intimate look into her thoughts and feelings during that initial acute phase of diagnosis and treatment. She shows us the coldly rational being, and the emotional and spiritual soul. She shows the interplay of family, friends, and faith in recovery; how zest for life and optimism affect treatment and outlook; and how a cancer victim brings laughter and love to what is otherwise a bleak and humorless picture.

Patty's story also tells of the great strides we have made in treating cancer. When viewed over the decades, the advances are amazing. You only have to go back to 1970 – one generation – to see these changes. In 1970, mammography was a new, unproven, and crude technique. In fact breast cancer treatment was virtually unchanged from the time of Dr. Roswell Park, one of the visionaries in cancer medicine at the turn of the last century. Virtually all women had radical mastectomy, with its severe disfigurement, pain, permanent impairment of the shoulder, and swelling of the arm. Nothing else was available. And even with this, most women eventually died from cancer that spread to other organs.

But in the '70s radical mastectomy gave way to radical change with the application of scientific method to cancer medicine. Research showed that radical mastectomy was not necessary, and the operation was relegated to history (I started surgical training in 1979 and never performed a radical mastectomy in training – for surgeons 5 years my senior, it was all they did). And building on these advances, subsequent research studies showed that removal of only the lump itself was needed, so that now we are able to treat most women without removing the breast.

Though mammography then provided crude, unfocused images by current standards, studies started in the 1970s showed that mammography could find small breast cancers that could not be felt as a lump. And the studies proved that mammography improves the odds of survival leading to the current recommendation that all women undergo periodic mammography.

Advances in understanding the biology of breast cancer led to the development of treatments that addressed the cancer cells that spread beyond the breast. Chemotherapy and anti-estrogen hormone drugs given after surgery were shown to actually cure many women who previously would have died from breast cancer with surgery alone. And recent studies showed that Tamoxifen, one of these anti-estrogen drugs, given to women at higher risk of breast cancer, actually reduces their chance of getting the disease in the first place.

Most importantly, work building on research of the last 30 years is revealing the secrets of cancer biology that will provide new approaches that will fundamentally change the way we approach this disease in the coming decades. There is now real reason to believe that the next generation, or perhaps the generation after that, will see cancer as a chronic, controllable disorder: we will be able to predict who will get it, to prevail in its treatment, and even to prevent it from occurring at all.

But Patty's story also sobers us with the many shortcomings and frustrations of breast cancer therapy.

- Despite the proven value of mammography, it did not help Patty. Hers was one of the 10% of breast cancers invisible to mammography. It was only found when she noticed a large lump in her armpit from breast cancer spread to lymph nodes. This is just the situation that we hope to prevent with screening mammography.

- Patty had to receive chemotherapy. We know that 60 to 70% of women with a cancer spread to the lymph nodes like Patty's actually have cancer spread to other organs, and that this cancer will eventually manifest itself, and result in death. But we have no way of determining who are among the 70% and who are not. Despite normal x-rays and scans showing no evidence of this spread, we know it has occurred, albeit in microscopic amounts, in most cases. The only option is to treat all of these women.

- Chemotherapy only helps some of the women who get it. It only reduces the chance of cancer recurrence, and ultimately of premature death, by about one-third. So in Patty's case, the chance of recurrence drops from, say, 60 to 70% to 40 to 45%. In the rest of the cases, the cancer cells survive the toxic chemotherapy drugs and continue growing. We cannot determine in which cases the cancer cells are susceptible to chemotherapy and in which they are not. Looked at another way, almost three-quarters of the women who receive chemotherapy for breast cancer gain nothing – either they weren't going to have cancer recurrence, or the chemotherapy doesn't prevent it. So while it may be life saving, and while women like Patty should take it, we must improve these therapies, and apply them only to those who benefit.

• We are unable to define who will get breast cancer. Patty assumed all her life that she would get it because of her family history. And though she did get cancer, testing for changes in the genes that we know are responsible for breast cancer in many families did not reveal a change in Patty. (We were surprised with this result because of her family history, and her ancestry – alterations in the common breast cancer genes occur more frequently in people of Ashkenazi Jewish ancestry.)

These shortcomings are not for want of looking for answers. Thousands of brilliant, dedicated people around the world have spent their entire careers trying to answer each of these questions. And they have made real progress. But we have a long way to go. This underscores the need for continued support for research in basic cancer biology and breast cancer treatment. It is only through this work that we will be able to resolve these questions and change the outlook for Patty's children and grandchildren.

On the personal level, I am grateful to Patty for providing insights into the art of medicine: how the treatment we provide and the counseling and support we administer are interpreted and used. Through her emails, she shows us how people blend personal values and experience in deciding what is best for them.

As an example, I was fascinated how she came to her decisions regarding mastectomy. Patty came to me for a second opinion, but seemed set to have both breasts removed. At the end of our first meeting, I thought she would proceed with this plan. I provided her the factual information that mastectomy would not affect her long-term odds of survival. Given the fact that she had a large lymph node under her armpit, and likely had other lymph nodes involved, the real risk to her life was that this cancer might have spread. Removing the breasts doesn't change this. The only rationale for removing one or both breasts is to prevent another breast cancer in the future. The potential of dying from that breast cancer pales in comparison to the real chance of early death from the known cancer. And surgery to remove both breasts is a big operation with real risks, to say nothing of its emotional impact. However, given her family history and concerns, it would be perfectly reasonable to have bilateral mastectomy.

Much to my surprise, the next day she called and asked that we proceed with lumpectomy if genetic testing did not show a change in the genes. She had this genetic testing, the test did not show any gene mutation, and we proceeded with lumpectomy. But her processing of the "data" was not so simple. Recent events suggest to me that time, events, and unwavering optimism have colored and molded that data. On a recent visit, she again raised the issue of removing both breasts. She rationalized that now that she had successfully completed chemotherapy, and was likely cured, that now was the time to proceed. While I again agreed it would be reasonable to do the mastectomies, I was forced to go right back to the first day and go through the data on the risk of cancer recurrence, the level of benefit she could see from chemotherapy, and the absence of benefit in this regard from the surgery.

I felt the pressures of my conflicting duties in her case to balance the sympathy I have for her situation and her belief that she has beat this cancer with the fact that further surgery at this point doesn't provide substantial help. I certainly felt the chilling effect of these facts on her that day. But surgery is not a treatment for her fears, and carries real immediate risks even beyond the pain and disability. However uncomfortable I feel for again forcing her to look at the hard facts, I also know from her emails that her inner force will provide her the strength, and that her love of life and others, and the love others have for her, will allow her to come to the decision that is best for her, and allow her to continue her full and happy life.

And ultimately, that is what I have learned from all the Pattys that I have served. People have a remarkable inner strength, a will to live, and an optimism that always conquers the darkness and pain they face. I stand in awe at the resilience and fortitude of people facing these diseases and their treatments. And I am grateful to Patty for sharing with us her struggle, and her strength. And through her, the strength of us all.

Acknowledgments

Thank you to all the people on my email list who responded to my missives with gratitude and support. Without their suggestions to turn the emails into some sort of publication, it would never have occurred to me to do so.

We appreciate the time and talent Leslie Zemsky donated to this project. Her enthusiasm encouraged me and her illustrations enhanced the book.

Thank you to the two members of my Park School of Buffalo family: Amy Greene, my friend since the fourth grade at Park, and Margaret Marcus, my former colleague when we taught together at Park in the '70s. They were my editors and tweaked the emails, turning my banter into a better book.

I have enjoyed working with Julianna Jacoby-Patronski, the coordinator of this project at Roswell Park Cancer Institute, and Beth Manos, our layout and design artist.

Thank you to my daughters, Sarah, Lisa, and Susan, and to my husband, Warren. They offered the perfect combination of curiosity, concern, and honest criticism.

About the Author

Patty Cohen Gelman graduated from the Park School of Buffalo in 1966 and from Boston University in 1970. She returned to Buffalo to teach Language Arts and Social Studies at Park School; married Warren Gelman in 1972; raised three daughters; and worked in the Development Office at Park as the Alumni Director. She currently is a volunteer fund-raiser for Park School, the Boys & Girls Clubs of Buffalo, and Roswell Park Cancer Institute in Buffalo.

****

We are grateful for the grants we received from several local foundations to publish this book.